RUNNING REPAIRS

A runner's guide to keeping injury free

Paula Coates

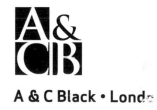

A & C Black • London

First published 2007 by
A & C Black Publishers Ltd
38 Soho Square, London W1D 3HB
www.acblack.com

Copyright © 2007

ISBN-13: 978 0 7136 8497 1

Note: It is always the responsibility of the individual to assess his or her own fitness capability before participating in any training activity. While every effort has been made to ensure the content of this book is as technically accurate as possible, neither the author nor the publishers can accept responsibility for any injury or loss sustained as a result of the use of this material.

Text and cover design © Mark Roberts at Talking Design
Cover photograph of runners in the 2006 Denver Marathon
© AP/Empics (Lyn Alweis)
Inside photographs courtesy of © Grant Pritchard, except p. 53 (Bananastock); pp. 31, 62, 79 (Digital Vision); pp. v, vi, 17 (Empics); pp. 52, 73, 74, 122 (istockphoto); pp. 18, 20, 22, 130 (Paula Coates) and p.33 (Photodisc).
Illustrations by Mark Silver

This book is produced using paper that is made from wood grown in managed, sustainable forests. It is natural, renewable and recyclable. The logging and manufacturing processes conform to the environmental regulations of the country of origin.

Typeset in Apex Sans Book
Printed and bound in China by Wing King Tong

›› CONTENTS

>> ACKNOWLEDGEMENTS

I would like to say a big thank you to all the people who have given their time and support to me during the writing of this book.

First and foremost to Robert Foss and Lucy Beevor at A&C Black, for their input and guidance throughout; to Annemarie O'Connor, musculoskeletal podiatrist, for her contribution and time spent proofreading the biomechanics section; to the members of Clapham Runners and others (including Dakota the dog, who was borrowed from her owner on Clapham Common) who have a starring role as models in the photos; to Balance physiotherapy for providing a location for the indoor photo shoot; and last but not least to Jane Burgess for her ideas and inspiration and to Ruth Boit for her encouragement over our many lunches!

My thanks also go to photographer Grant Pritchard and to Graham Marsh who introduced me to Robert Foss.

Finally, I must thank all my patients who have inspired me to write this book. Happy running, and I hope I can help you stay injury free.

Paula Coates

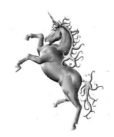

›› INTRODUCTION

There is a certain look that has become very familiar to me. I see it all the time on the faces of people visiting my physiotherapy clinic – although it tends to be more common from January to March, when training for the spring marathon season is in full swing. The look says, 'I'm injured, so my running days are over' and it's exactly the same on the person trying to get in shape for their first 5km fun run as it is for the seasoned marathon runner who has a personal best firmly in their sights.

My response always starts in the same way, with the words 'Don't look so worried, it's almost certainly not as bad as you think.' Then I explain that I have clocked up five marathon finishes and know the highs and lows that go with the territory. If they take my advice and don't try too much too soon – that's always the hard bit to stick to – they will be back in their trainers in no time. There is a look of relief, an easing of tension in the shoulders, and we're ready to start treating the injury.

As a runner – no matter what standard you perceive yourself to be – you are in a select group of the population: somewhere in the top 10 per cent or so of the most active people in the country, in fact. Good for you! Not only are you physically active, but the chances are that you keep an eye on what you eat and drink and generally take good care of yourself. The training that you do may come with the odd injury setback now and again, and there will be times when you just don't fancy going for that run, but overall your training is making you a stronger, fitter, healthier and happier person. Think about that for a minute, as it's easy to forget when you're constantly pushing yourself for this distance or that time, or balancing a hectic life in order to get one or two runs in a week.

A good proportion of the runners that turn up to my clinic don't need to be there. Now, I'm not trying to put myself out of work – there are times when you must seek specialist help and advice – and the skills of a physiotherapist are worth every penny. I will make this very clear throughout the book. However, with some careful planning and appropriate training you should be able to avoid most of the injuries that plague us as runners. Should you pick up the odd ache or pain – and we all do at some point – then self-treatment is often the most effective way to start. That's why I've written this book.

As a runner, when I'm training for a particular race I seem to exist in one of three states: injured; recovering from injury; or wondering where the next injury will come from. It needn't be this way. My aim here as a physiotherapist is to put injury into perspective so that it's just one more item on the list of runners' concerns – just like what colour top to run in, what new gadget to go for, how to justify biscuits in the name of carb-loading, that sort of thing.

The book is split into three main parts. **Part 1** covers the basics. If you think of your body as a machine, then this section is the instruction manual that you would read before using it for the first time. There are a couple of problems with this approach. Your body isn't brand new, alas, and most people never take the instructions out of the box, let alone

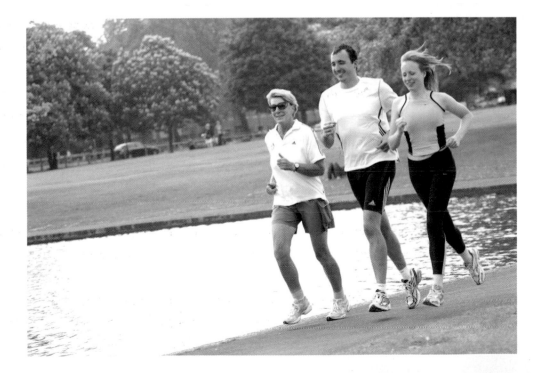

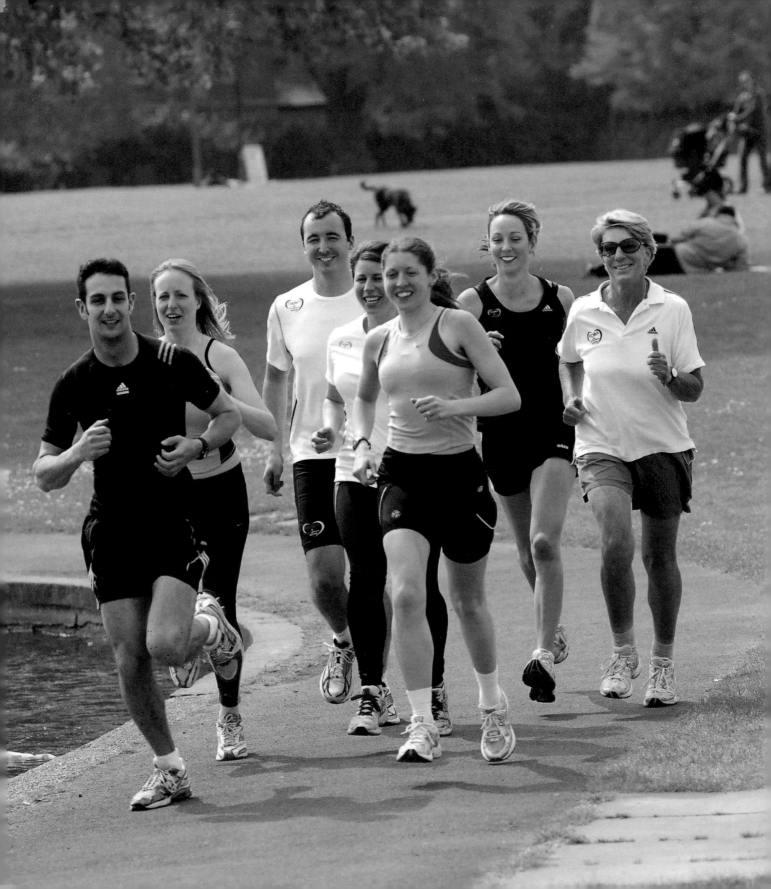

read them. But do take the time to look at this section. It will help you to understand how your body works and what happens when you run. It also covers some of the other things that you need to think about when getting started, such as buying the right kit and shoes. I've also included some tips on how to start your return from an injury – remember, not too much too soon. It finishes up with your very own MOT and service history; by answering a few questions about yourself, you should get a good idea of the type of runner you are, and this will highlight potential injury hotspots for you to work on before they cause a problem.

Part 2 looks at 'the usual suspects'. These are the villains of the piece – boo, hiss! This section lists the most common injuries that runners are likely to come across, so that you can work out what you have done to yourself. This in no way replaces an assessment with your physiotherapist but it will help you understand what you may have done and why it has happened. It will teach you how to manage the acute phase of each injury, as well as answering some of the questions you may have about what happens next.

Part 3 covers repair and prevention. We all know that prevention is better than cure, even if it's not always the most pleasant thing in the world – I still remember my TB vaccination when I was a child. This section is the runner's vaccination. It includes all the stretches and exercises that will help you to avoid injury in the first place, or help you to come back fitter and stronger from an injury lay-off. You may dismiss them when all you want to do – or have time for – is to get out there and run, but I promise you that minutes spent on these exercises will keep you on your feet for longer, overall, and will even improve your fitness and times. Just take a deep breath and add them to your training – you will learn to love these sessions when you see the results.

> **>> FITNESS FACT**
>
> Make running injury-free your ultimate goal. That way you will achieve all your other goals.

This book first came to my mind in 2005. With just six weeks to go until the London Marathon, I badly sprained my ankle. I looked at my schedule and it didn't say 'stop training for two weeks' – the schedules never say that, do they? I wracked my brain for solutions. I even dragged my podiatrist – who fortunately is a good friend – over to my clinic at 9am on a Sunday morning just in case she could do something I hadn't already thought of myself. A little overdramatic, maybe, but that's how much it meant to me at the time. It wasn't until I was running over Tower Bridge and turning right along the highway six weeks later that it dawned on me why I had got back into training so quickly with minimal impact on my fitness. I was lucky in that I had had professional knowledge at my fingertips. Having that expertise to hand was the difference between making the start line and watching the race on TV. This knowledge is exactly what runners need in order to prevent and manage their injuries. There are many questions that you ask yourself when you are injured, and having the answers at hand will speed up your recovery and prevent injury in the future.

So, if you're fit and well then make sure you read Part 1 so that you stay that way. If you're suffering with an injury, look it up, find out what to do and, most importantly of all, don't worry. Happy running!

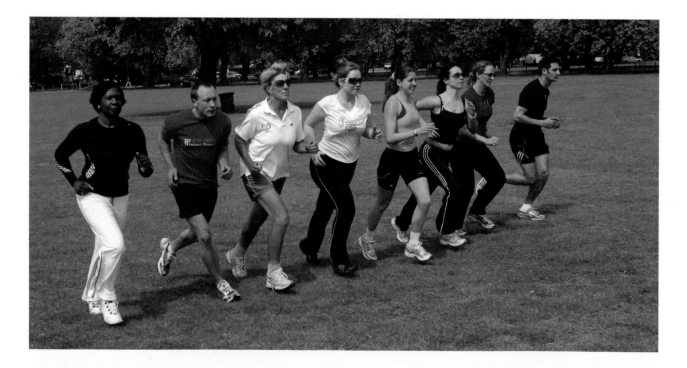

Note: throughout Part 3 there are case studies to illustrate the prevention and cure strategies used to treat running injuries. Use this chart to find the most relevant case studies for you.

Case study	Sex	Age	Condition	Page no.
1	Male	42	Neck pain	118
2	Male	35	Low-back pain	126
3	Female	26	Buttock pain (Piriformis syndrome)	128
4	Female	42	Hip and thigh pain	135
5	Female	32	Post-natal incontinence	137
6	Male	58	Knee pain	141
7	Female	25	Thigh pain	144
8	Male	32	Achilles pain	149
9	Female	25	Foot pain	153
10	Male	34	Shin pain	157

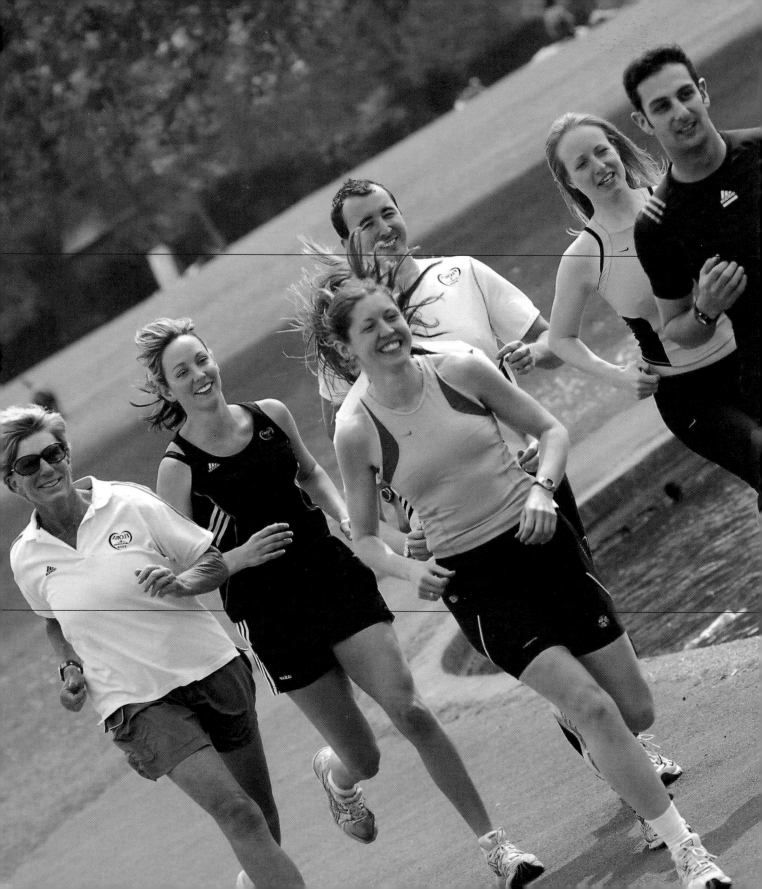

1

THE ESSENTIALS

This part of the book is all about getting to know yourself. If you understand how your body moves when you run, you'll be able to train to your strengths, manage possible areas of weakness and pick the best kit to support you. If you think of your body as a machine, then this is your very own MOT. We're going to see how you've looked after your engine in the past – what sort of mileage you've done, and whether you're more used to long journeys on the motorway or the occasional trip to the local shop. Then we're going to put you through a full service to see what sort of shape all the moving parts are in at the moment. By the time you're at the end of Part 1, you'll be finely tuned and ready for the road.

CONTENTS

YOUR BODY BIOMECHANICS

Having a basic understanding of how your body works will help you to manage an injury. You'll know who can give you the best professional advice and when to visit them. It can also help you to train properly to avoid injury in the first place (more details in Part 3).

When it comes to pinpointing specific biomechanical patterns or running styles that cause injury, it is fair to assume that an individual with an abnormal or inefficient running style is more likely to suffer injury. A variety of anatomical anomalies are blamed for the development of overuse-type injuries, which commonly lead to specific aches and pains. Overpronation, for example, can predispose you to medial tibial stress syndrome (shin splints) or bow legs, leading to iliotibial band syndrome (see page 78). However, it is not true that all runners who overpronate, or are bow-legged, will definitely suffer these injuries; issues related to training errors are often more to blame.

WHAT WILL INFLUENCE YOUR RUNNING BIOMECHANICS?

The following factors can all affect your running biomechanics:

- posture
- leg alignment (knock-knees or bow legs)
- foot anomalies (pronation or supination)
- range of movement at all your joints
- muscle imbalances
- flexibility
- pelvic instability
- neuromuscular firing patterns
- leg length discrepancies

All these factors sound complex, but in reality they are not. Your posture, leg alignment and foot type are down to genetics and body type. All the factors are influenced by the flexibility of your joints and muscles and how in balance this is with the way you use your body. Neuromuscular firing patterns are dictated by repetition and use, so the more you do something the more likely you are to have a firing pattern that performs an activity in a certain way.

Pelvic instability and leg length discrepancies are commonly used phrases, but they don't mean that your pelvis or leg is structurally unstable. Instead, they refer to how your muscles control (or don't control) the movement around your pelvis and spine. It is common to have one leg slightly longer than the other, and this isn't always a problem – it's just the way you are, and some professional footballers even use it to their advantage. Some people will benefit from a heel raise to alter a discrepancy, but some won't. If you're worried, speak to your chartered physiotherapist or podiatrist.

Every runner has their own tolerance to the stresses of running and it will take a combination of factors to cause a runner's body to pass that threshold and into injury. So don't let your knock knees or flat feet stop you from running, just make sure you train properly and wear the correct trainers!

HOW DO YOU RUN?

Very few runners fit the mechanical ideal, so it is unlikely that you will be one of them. The best way to find out how you run is to get someone to record you (this is easily done as most digital cameras and even mobile phones have a video recording capacity). I often video people running and compare images of them in different styles of running shoe and when barefoot. This is the easiest way to demonstrate the effects a shoe can have on the position of the whole leg when you are running. It is also a great way to record improvements before and after injury and rehabilitation.

If you are recording yourself, make particular note of the following factors:

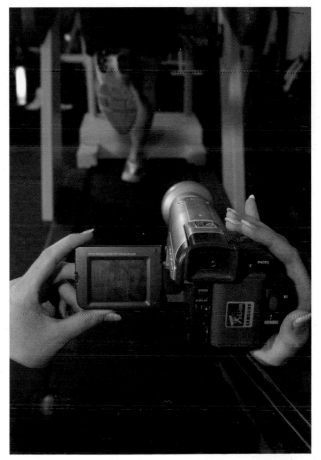

- Are your shoulders relaxed? If not, relax them.
- What are your arms doing? Try to keep your elbows at a 90-degree angle. Focus on the backward swing, then let your arms come forward and half-way across your body.
- Do you have knock knees? If so, can you change this by altering your running style?
- What kind of foot striker are you? Check which part of your foot hits the ground first when you run without shoes. This will help you to decide which trainers are best for you.
- Run with your trainers on. Do you look any different from the way you run barefoot?
- Do you lean forward or are you very upright? A slight forward lean is good; try it and see how it feels.
- Can you hear your footfall? Is it heavy and loud? Can you make it quieter? Does this look and feel different?

Ideally, you should record yourself at regular intervals (say, every four to six months) to monitor your training progress and to keep an eye on areas of potential weakness. If possible, it is also a good idea to record yourself at different stages of a run (for example, when you are fresh as well as towards the end of a long run when you start to fatigue and poor form starts to creep in) and at different speeds. You will need a good, patient friend to do the recording. The easiest place to do this is on a treadmill, as the recorder will be able to focus on you without worrying about moving themself. However, it is good to get outside as your running style will change subtly when on a treadmill.

Before going into what to look for in your videos (see 'The Camera Never Lies' on page 12), we need to get a grasp of how your body is supposed to work when you run.

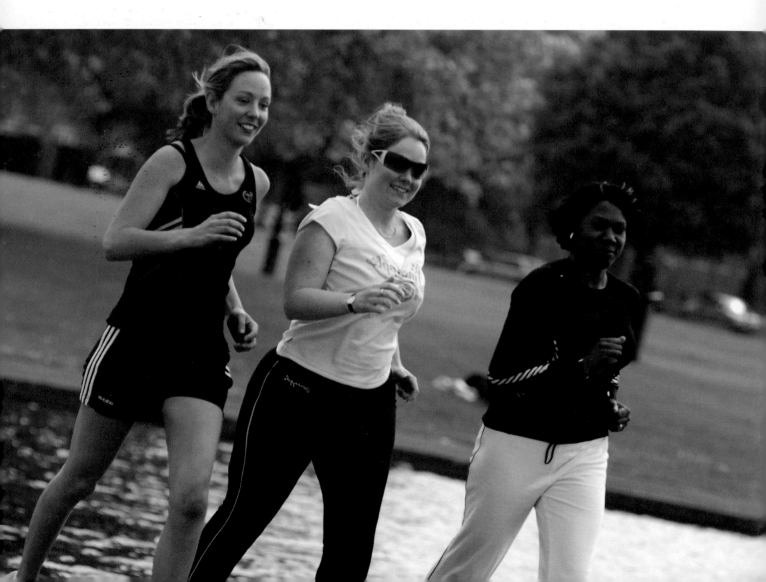

STABILITY AND MOBILITY

By its very nature, running is an unstable activity, with alternate landing on one leg and then the other. At one stage both feet are off the ground at once. Therefore, the key to avoiding injury is to ensure that you improve your stability and mobility in the key areas that contribute to running mechanics. These areas are, from head to toe:

- **arms and upper body** – the key to this area is mobility and symmetry which allows free and equal movement of the arms to support propulsion (forward movement)
- **lower back and core** – muscle strength is needed here to provide stability to help with pelvic and hip alignment
- **hips** – mobility and flexibility is the order of the day, again to allow a full and controlled range of movement of the legs
- **knees** – the knee is a critical joint and stability is vital in order to control the forces and movement that go with running
- **ankles and feet** – controlled mobility is required to allow your body to react to changes in the running surface, to achieve the best possible foot strike position and to aid propulsion.

From this you can see there is a clear relationship between the various areas of the body: mobility-stability-control-mobility-stability-flexibility. We will return to this throughout the book, as well as looking at each of these areas in more detail in this section. But for now, the main point is that time spent on developing functional strength – which is an area often overlooked in a runner's training programme – will help to maintain controlled alignment and flexibility in your legs, especially if you are not genetically blessed with fantastic biomechanics. This can prevent many niggles and injuries.

> **>> FITNESS FACT**
>
> Seventy per cent of injuries are due to training errors, including the amount of running and sudden changes in speed and distance.

> **>> FITNESS FACT**
>
> Make sure you are safe when you run. Avoid dark and unlit areas, carry a mobile phone and leave details of when you left and when you will be back.

THE RUNNING CYCLE

Running is basically alternating hops from left to right leg with a bit of forward movement thrown in and some upward lift from the arms. Looking at it a bit more technically, the 'running cycle', as it is known, is made up of four distinct phases (see fig. 1.1):

1. **Contact** – when one foot is on the ground.
2. **Propulsion** – the final push through the toes before the leg swings forward.
3. **Float** – where both legs are off the ground.
4. **Swing** – when the leg not contacting the floor is swinging forward.

Contact

Initial contact is when the foot first touches the ground. It is important to know which type of striker you are as this will have a great effect on the rest of your running mechanics. For example:

- **Heel strikers** will hit the ground with their heel first, and have a tendency to overstride. Impact through the foot and knee is greater, which may make you more prone to injury and will wear out your trainers more quickly.

STRIKE STYLE

Remember, everyone is different so, before you change your strike style, think about the following:

- If you are not getting injured, do you need to change your style? If it's not broken, don't fix it!
- It takes time to learn and then improve speed and time with a new style.
- The correct trainers will help to support your natural running style, so review this first.
- Ask a biomechanical expert to look at your style before embarking on a change regime.

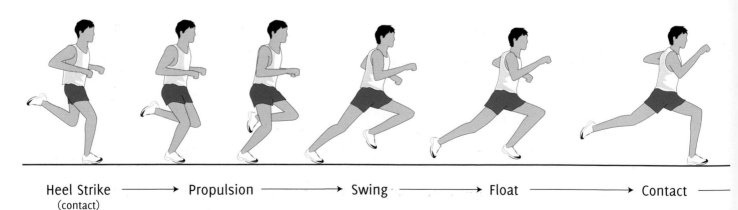

Heel Strike ⟶ Propulsion ⟶ Swing ⟶ Float ⟶ Contact ⟶
(contact)

Fig 1.1: The running cycle

- **Mid-foot strikers** demonstrate a more natural style and will be less noisy when running on a treadmill. They will experience less shock to the tissues of the lower leg. It is also a more efficient way to run, so less energy is used. This can mean quicker speeds over distance for less perceived effort.
- **Forefoot strikers** are the natural sprinters of the pack. This is good over shorter and middle distances, but not ideal for a marathon!

As I mentioned before, taking a video is a great way of analysing your running, but you can also make a reasonable judgement as to what type of striker you are by the wear on the soles of your trainers. Remember that walking is typically a heel-strike activity, so if you walk a lot in your trainers this may cause them to wear at the heel more.

Your body controls the landing with your knee and ankle flexing and your foot rolling in (pronating). It is during the contact phase that you are at the greatest risk of injury. This is because your muscles are controlling the position of the joints and the stability of the leg while absorbing the impact of the foot striking the ground. It is the repetition of the inability to control a good leg position that leads to injury. Knowing how you run and where you are lacking functional strength will help you to calculate which of the strength, conditioning and stretching exercises in Part 3 will help you the most. Thinking about each part of your body as you run is a good way to monitor relaxation, maintain a good arm swing and keep to a good style; this is particularly helpful as you fatigue. It will also help you to refocus and keep good form. This is the perfect time to think about which type of foot striker you are. If you run on a treadmill you can listen to how noisy you are; by making less noise you will reduce the impact on your legs.

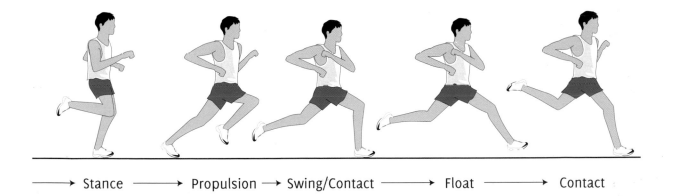

Stance ⟶ Propulsion ⟶ Swing/Contact ⟶ Float ⟶ Contact

Propulsion

Propulsion is the point at which the foot leaves the ground and the toes push off to take the leg forward towards the next step. The ankle, knee and hip all extend (straighten) to push the body upwards and forwards. This phase uses energy that has been stored in the tendons and muscles during the absorption of impact in the initial contact phase. During propulsion, try to think about pushing off through the big toe. This will help to keep the ankle joint in a stable, supinated position and prevent you from rolling your ankle, which can occur if you are tired or if you push through your other toes.

Float

This phase is what separates walking from running – it is the moment when neither foot is in contact with the ground. Technically, there is no risk at this stage, but impact is not far away.

Swing

The swing phase begins immediately after propulsion when the foot, positioned in preparation for weight bearing, is carried forward to strike the ground and the muscles stabilising the body prepare to absorb the impact of contact. Once the foot strikes the ground, the swing phase ends and a new cycle begins. The main thing to focus on during this phase is lifting the knee to drive the leg forward. Runners with a lazy or low leg swing are more likely to trip up; this is also a common problem with fatigue. The best way to improve your swing is to perform more hill runs, either outside or on the treadmill, as you can't help but lift your knees when running uphill.

UPPER BODY AND ARM MECHANICS

The main function of the upper body and arm action when running is to provide balance and encourage momentum. During the contact phase, the arms and trunk produce a propulsive force and can be used to assist forward momentum. During distance running, the normal arm action involves pulling the shoulder and elbow back, then, as the arm comes forward, the hand moves slightly across the body. Arm action is more important for running efficiency than injury prevention. Equal arm action can also contribute to vertical lift and speed during propulsion, which may help runners to be more efficient and reduce the work done by the legs.

> **>> FITNESS FACT**
>
> Concentrate on your posture and running technique rather than your time and pace. It gives you something useful to think about!

PELVIS AND TRUNK MECHANICS

When the foot makes contact with the ground, the trunk should ideally be flexed forwards 5–10 degrees and the pelvis tipped forwards 15–20 degrees. During the contact phase – when impact is absorbed – trunk flexion will increase as the pelvis tilt remains stable. This position of the trunk helps to maintain the body's forward and horizontal momentum. The gluteals, hamstrings, abdominals and back muscles are all involved in controlling the trunk and pelvis during this phase.

During propulsion, the trunk extends back to the same position as during initial contact. The pelvic tilt, however, will increase. This helps to direct the propulsion force of the leg to move the body horizontally and forwards.

ANKLE, KNEE AND HIP MECHANICS

The muscles controlling the ankle, knee and hip work together to provide propulsion upwards and forwards throughout the running cycle. These muscles work in unison to provide an energy-efficient mechanism for running. During the contact phase, the activity of the calf, quadriceps, hamstring and gluteal muscles is lower than during propulsion. This reduced activity is possible because the muscles of the foot and the Achilles tendon have the ability to store energy during the contact phase which they can release later in the cycle, during the propulsion phase. It is therefore important to train specifically to strengthen your legs to absorb and control impact while maintaining an efficient running style. Functional strength training that is specific to running helps you to control the position of your legs and prevents the hip and knee rolling in.

Rotational control from the hip, knee and foot is crucial in injury prevention. Having a mid-foot strike reduces the impact and loading of the joints and muscles, but doesn't prevent injury. Because mid-foot strikers flex more at the knee and ankle than heel or forefoot strikers, they have a greater ability to absorb impact forces throughout the leg rather than through foot pronation alone. However, in order to make the most of their running strike, they must train as much as anyone else to improve rotational strength control throughout the whole leg.

Eccentric strength training in the calf and quadriceps muscles is essential to control the knee and ankle joints. Eccentric strength refers to situations where the muscle works as it lengthens. When running, eccentric muscle action can be likened to a breaking action, as it slows movement and controls the position of the joints. It is more common to think of a muscle becoming short and fat when it is active, but it is important for muscles to be able to work as they lengthen as well. Without this function, the knee and ankle would collapse or rotate inwards during running.

Good runners will use efficient muscle action and movement patterns. It is essential that the ankle and knee can quickly control the forces involved in running and create a stable leg. This is where good technique is vital. Too much upward bounce increases the force when you land, putting greater impact on the joints and requiring more muscle strength to control the forces acting on the leg. At slower running speeds, these forces can be two to three times bodyweight. As a runner, it is important to learn to bounce forwards rather than upwards by taking quick, light steps.

Excessive impact or breaking forces can contribute to injury. The correct movement patterns of the hip, knee and ankle alongside correct activation and strength of the leg muscles will help to control braking forces during running, resulting in a more efficient action using elastic energy stored in the tendons and minimising landing forces. Heel strikers tend to keep their knee relatively straighter on contact and absorb impact by foot rotation (pronation), while mid-foot and forefoot strikers will tend to keep the knee and foot flexed, absorbing impact in a more elastic fashion.

FOOT MECHANICS

Pronation seems to be the word on every runner's lips – get two or more of us in a room and within two minutes someone will have said the word. However, it is widely misunderstood and it is worth spending a few minutes clearing things up.

(a)	(b)	(c)

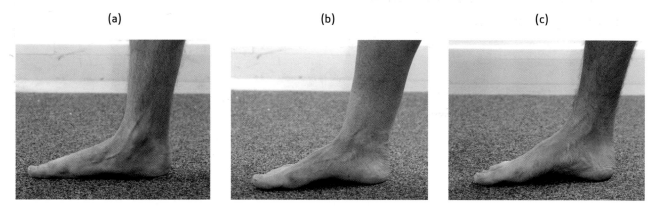

Fig. 1.2 The three types of foot strike: (a) pronation, (b) neutral and (c) supination

Inward and outward rolling of the foot during running are called pronation and supination, respectively. This rolling action is normal – it is only excessive pronation or supination that can lead to injury. It is important to run with a running style that is natural to you and to use the correct trainers or orthotics to support your foot posture (see pages 18–22). You can also affect what happens at the foot by making changes to your posture and strengthening your pelvis. In addition, you can improve your ability and move towards becoming a midfoot striker, thus reducing the impact forces through the leg, by increasing your pelvic tilt.

An excessive supinator will lose out on the shock-absorbing benefits of normal pronation movements. Excessive supinators tend to suffer from injuries to the lateral knee and hip, and can also be prone to stress fractures because of the higher repetitive impact forces.

Excessive pronators tend to suffer from anterior knee pain, medial tibial stress syndrome, Achilles tendon and soft-tissue injuries around the foot and and ankle.

Wet footprints

One simple and useful way to get an idea of your foot strike and pronation tendencies is to look at your footprint. When you next take a shower, walk across a flat, even and dry surface and take a look at the footprint you leave behind. This will tell you whether you have high- or low-arched feet (see fig. 1.3).

1. Toes and forefoot plus heel, joined by a broad band – indicates a neutral foot strike.
2. Entire foot – indicates low or flat arches which are associated with overpronation.
3. Toes plus heels, but with little in between – indicates high arches which are associated with excessive supination.

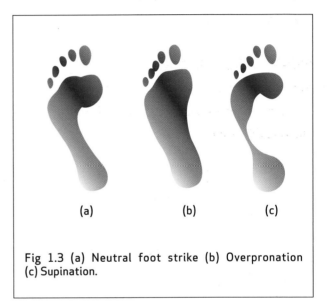

(a)   (b)   (c)

Fig 1.3 (a) Neutral foot strike (b) Overpronation (c) Supination.

THE CAMERA NEVER LIES

Looking at your posture when you are running can tell you a lot about your muscles. Listed below are some of the areas for improvement that I regularly spot in runners.

The domino effect

Too much forward lean (see fig. 1.4) suggests that the hamstrings, gluteals and spinal muscles are weak, increasing the risk of a strain on the hamstrings and back . Fix it by using:

- Hamstring curls (see page 142)
- Leg circles (see page 132)
- Bridges (see page 129)

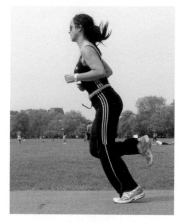

Fig. 1.4 Forward lean

The pogo stick

If your posture is too upright (see fig. 1.5) it encourages vertical instead of forward movement, which increases landing forces, slowing your pace. This makes you prone to injury and stress fractures. Fix it by:

- Increasing your stride length (this will take practice)
- Making your running quieter on the treadmill
- Using the crucifix stretch (see page 125)
- Using the dynamic hamstring stretch (see page 146)

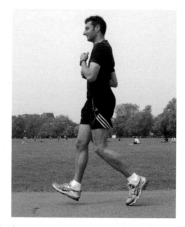

Fig. 1.5 Posture too upright

Does my bum look big in this?

Too much forward tilt at the pelvis (see fig. 1.6) indicates weakness in the gluteals and abdominals, which means control of the pelvis during landing is poor. It may also suggest tight hip flexors. Fix it by using :

- Cossack stretch (see page 133)
- Walking lunges (see page 143)

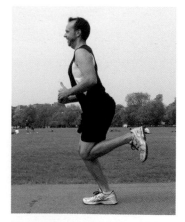

Fig. 1.6 Too much forward tilt at the pelvis

Bum? What bum?

An excessive anterior pelvic tilt during the propulsion phase (see fig. 1.7) could be a sign of tight hip flexors and a reduced range of movement when the hip is extending. This reduces drive from the hip and can cause low-back pain. It is common to have a flat bum and less of a curve in your low back if you run like this. Fix by using:

- Walking lunges (see page 143)
- One-legged stepper (see page 130)

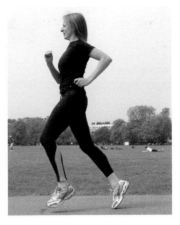

Fig. 1.7 Excessive tilt at the pelvis during propulsion

The duck

A poor trunk position, or lack of pelvic stability (see fig. 1.8) can reduce the efficiency of the running action, creating extra load on the leg muscles or increasing stress through the lumbar spine and pelvis. It may also allow the knee of the stance leg to rotate inwards, which can increase the pronation forces on the ankle. All could lead to injury. Fix by:

- Wearing good trainers
- Seeing a physiotherapist
- Using all of the exercises in Part 3

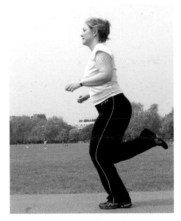

Fig. 1.8 Poor trunk position or lack of pelvic stability

The hip-wiggler

The gluteals, quadratus lumborum and abdominal muscles are of primary importance in providing lateral stability of the whole leg (see Fig. 1.9). They contract prior to and during the contact phase, preventing the hip from dropping down too far on the side of the swinging leg. The muscles will be acting with gravity as well as against it to prevent this movement. You might get aches and pains around the low back and hips which can become a problem. Piriformis syndrome is common as the muscle becomes tight and overactive. Fix by using:

- Hip dips (see page 131)
- Leg circles (see page 132)

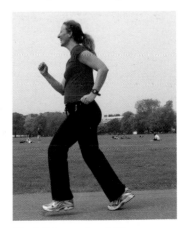

Fig. 1.9 Lateral stability

IT'S ALL IN THE STYLE

Hopefully, the brief overview of the running cycle and basic biomechanics above has given you some food for thought. The intention is not for every runner to adopt the 'ideal' style – it's just not possible, as we all have our unique traits. Rather, by understanding how you run and how the various parts of your body interact to get you moving forwards, you should be consciously focusing on areas that affect you specifically while you run, developing a functional strength training programme to address any problem areas.

You should also be able to see the clear relationship between biomechanics and injury. Poor mechanics increase the landing forces acting on the body and thus the work that needs to be done by the muscles. Both increase stress on the body, which – depending on the individual and the amount of running undertaken – can cause injury.

So, we can sum up an individual's biomechanics quite simply: good technique and running style improves performance. So, when you are next out for your run, give some thought to the following factors:

- stride length and rate
- increased knee flexion during the swing phase
- slight forward lean when running
- increased plantarflexion (toes pointing) during propulsion
- sufficient arm swing across the body
- maintaining a narrow base of support.

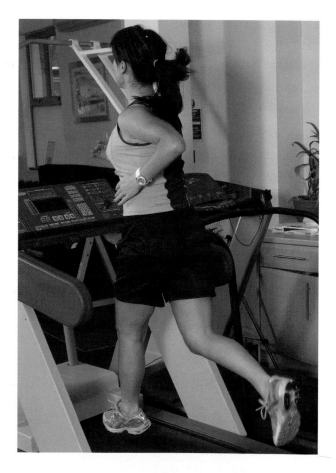

Your stride length and rate should be steady and even, which will enable you to judge your pace more accurately and help maintain good form. As I have mentioned before, lifting your knees during the swing phase and pushing off from your big toe is important. Think about propulsion and swing together: imagine pointing your toes behind you as you lift your knee along an invisible slope in front of you – the swing of the arms on the backward swing will help you to lift your leg up that slope before putting your foot in front of you. When thinking about the best amount of forward lean for running, take care to get the balance right. Lean forward enough to avoid the 'pogo stick'

posture and allow you to maintain momentum, but don't adopt the domino effect posture. Maintaining a narrow base of support is tricky and is dictated by the width of your hips (sorry ladies), but imagining that you have to stay in lane on a track will help you to focus on a narrow base. Take time to get to know how you run and you will save yourself a lot of bother later.

RUNNING METHODS

Before we leave the world of biomechanics, it is worth mentioning one or two of the current popular running 'methods'. Most of us don't really think about how we run; to borrow the well-known slogan, we 'just do it'. However, good technique can and does make a difference to efficiency, performance and injury prevention. If you are keen to go beyond the basics of the running cycle, then there are many books and countless courses on different running methods. Here is some background on two – chosen not because they are better than the others, just because they seem to be enjoying considerable popularity at the moment.

Pose running

No, this technique doesn't mean you need to spend loads of money on fancy new kit. Pose running was invented by Nicholas Romanov, a Russian scientist and consultant to the British, US and Mexican triathlon associations. During the 1970s–80s, he was heavily involved with training athletes in Russia. He noticed that his athletes would start to get injured as their workload increased. At this time, there was little focus on strength and conditioning training or underlying running technique, and heavy emphasis on mileage and speed training.

Romanov proposed a universal technique for all runners, regardless of speed or distance. The pose running technique is designed to prevent undue strain on the joints and requires a great deal of muscular endurance and resilience. According to Romanov, the Ethiopian distance champion Haile Gebrselassie and the US sprint legend Michael Johnson are both examples of runners with a natural pose style who were born with perfect technique.

The concept is simple enough, but in practice it is extremely hard to master. The distinguishing characteristic of this technique is that the athlete lands on the mid-foot, with the supporting joints flexed at impact, and then uses the hamstring muscles to pull the foot from the ground, relying on gravity to propel the runner forward. It is in clear contrast to the more common heel-strike method. Running should be easy, effortless, smooth and flowing. The runner should fall forwards, changing support from one leg to the other by pulling the foot from the ground. The pose running technique is centred on the idea that a runner maintains a single pose or position, moving continually forwards in this position.

Pose is by no means accepted by everybody in the running fraternity or backed up by sound scientific research. It is possible that many of the benefits of pose running are the result of rigorous strengthening programmes that are part of the training drills Romanov prescribes.

THE POSE TECHNIQUE ...

- maximises the use of gravity and minimises braking
- allows the leg to drop to the ground, touching down with the mid-foot of the supporting leg directly under the hip
- uses the hamstrings to pull the leg back into extension under the hip
- ensures that the hips are not pulled forward or pushed back
- uses arm movement for balance rather than force production
- maintains a high cadence.

Barefoot running

The idea of walking or running barefoot is a new concept only if you live in the western world. In India, Africa, China and Mexico it is commonplace; it is also popular in cross-country events in Queensland, Australia. However, the idea is now being taken up in the West and a new wave of barefoot runners aim to challenge the medical establishment and the way most of us run. As with the pose method, the technique lacks detailed scientific research at this stage, but it has been associated with substantially fewer acute injuries in the developing world – although this could be due to fewer injuries being reported or fewer runners seeking treatment.

Before you jump to the conclusion that this is just another trendy fad, it is worth remembering some well-known international athletes who were barefoot runners:

- **Zola Budd-Pieterse** – ran for South Africa, twice World Champion in 5km and cross-country
- **Abebe Bikila** – won Olympic gold in the marathon for Ethiopia in the 1960 Games
- **Herb Elliot** – won Olympic gold in 1960 in the 1500m, and also achieved 17 sub-four-minute miles.

Barefoot runners claim that running in shoes blocks communication from the outside world to the feet and body, and there may be some support for this idea. There are thousands of specialised receptors in the feet, which are designed to send messages to the brain via the central nervous system. The messages are interpreted by the brain and spinal cord, which then send back a command through motor response to the muscles. This allows us to react and move in a co-ordinated way, constantly adapting to changes in posture and the ground. Research shows that wearing trainers reduces the amount of information taken in, diminishing quality of movement and possibly leading to injury. The effect is likened to wearing gloves all day – think about how that would affect your ability to perform everyday tasks with your hands.

At the biomechanical level, this technique does seem to promote good practice:

- the bare foot naturally lands in more of a mid-foot position
- flexion at the ankle and knee is increased, which reduces impact (the body's natural break)
- sensory feedback from the soles of the feet is increased
- there is increased intrinsic muscle work, which builds strength in the foot.

There must be something to this approach, as many of the major sports shoe brands are trying to get in on the act (which I guess they would, as a world of barefoot runners would be a tricky place for a sports shoe manufacturer!). For example, Nike's Free range is intended to replicate many of the benefits of barefoot running while giving the foot some protection.

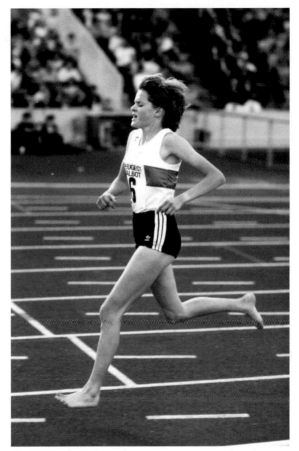
Fig 1.10 Zola Budd

TIPS FOR BAREFOOT RUNNING

- Start walking before running and build up slowly to allow the skin to gain its natural protective layer.
- Begin on grass or softer surfaces.
- Watch where you walk/run to avoid injury.
- If you feel aching around the smaller bones of your foot, stop barefoot running until the aching has completely gone to avoid stress fractures.
- Add a barefoot run on the treadmill to your training.

YOUR TRAINERS

If I were allowed to give you just one piece of advice in the whole book, it would be this: make sure you have the right pair of running shoes. There is no make or model that is best, but there is a make and model that is best for you. Buying the trainers that suit your individual running style and the distance you plan to run is incredibly important. You don't have to buy the most expensive, but you will need to pay £60 at the very least.

Good running shoes have the ability to absorb shock and guide your foot through its natural movement, and consequently have an important role to play in injury prevention. In fact, they have a role to play in every part of the running cycle:

- **Contact** – a dense, cushioned mid-sole will reduce impact forces in the heel and the forefoot.
- **Propulsion** – the style and location of the grooves in the sole will assist and guide the flexibility in the forefoot.
- **Float** – the lighter the shoe, the less you have to lift and carry through swing phase.
- **Swing** – again, a lighter shoe requires less effort to carry through the swing phase, and this will help to increase your pace.

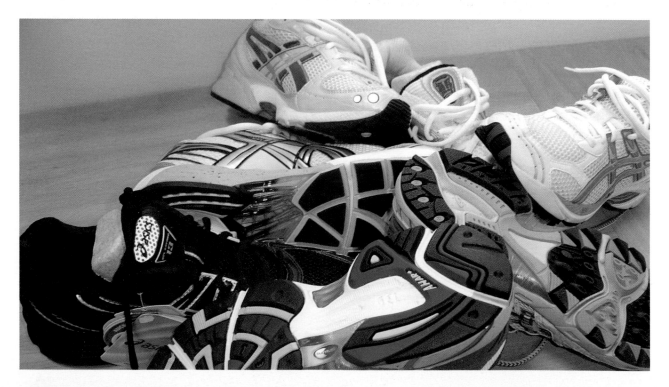

GOING SHOPPING

With running increasing in popularity as a way of keeping fit, specialist running shops can be found in most major towns and cities – and, with so much at stake, it really is worth going to one of these shops to buy your trainers. Don't be tempted to pick up a bargain online, and certainly don't buy the first pair of cross-trainers you see in your average high-street sports shop. I promise you that trying to pick out a bargain when it comes to trainers is a false economy – not only could it lead to injury but, if it does, you will have to bin the trainers and get a proper pair anyway.

Different shops will have different ways of assessing your feet and your running style: some will get you to try pairs out on a treadmill and video your feet; some will ask you to run across a pad on the floor connected to a computer, which creates an image of the impact regions on your feet; and some will simply watch you running up and down the pavement in different pairs of trainers. All of these are perfectly valid methods, so long as the person assessing you knows what to look for.

They should also ask you a few questions, such as:
- Do you have a history of injury?
- What size shoe are you? (They will probably measure this and may recommend a slightly larger size than you are used to, as feet tend to swell when you run over longer distances.)
- How many miles/hours a week do you intend to run?
- How heavy are you?
- Do you wear othotics?

It may also be worth taking your old trainers with you as these can often provide some tell-tale signs of your running style. Finally, don't be afraid to ask questions. Specialist shops are a great place to get top tips – the staff are usually keen runners and they see countless people pursuing the same dream as you.

>> **FITNESS FACT**

- Buy the right shoes for you. Always get properly assessed and buy for function not fashion.
- Don't put running shoes in the washing machine.

TYPES OF SHOE

When you are looking at running shoes you will generally see them described in one of four ways:

1. Motion control – very firm control and prevention of overpronation.

2. Stability – limits overpronation, but less so than motion control trainers.

3. Neutral – for runners who have an ideal biomechanical foot type and don't require control from their shoe.

4. Supinator/cushioned – for runners who have a heavy foot strike at the heel or forefoot but do not overpronate.

You will also see different shoes for different events and situations, for example trail shoes for off-road running and lightweight race shoes for shorter distances.

You don't need to worry about this bewildering array of choice, as the answers to the questions listed on page 19 and observation of your running style should lead the shop assistant to make most of the choices for you.

REAR-FOOT LACING

Try re-tying your laces (see fig. 1.11). It's a small tip, but will make your foot feel more secure in your trainers. It also lets you make the most of the structure and cushioning of the sole, no matter which type of shoe you wear.

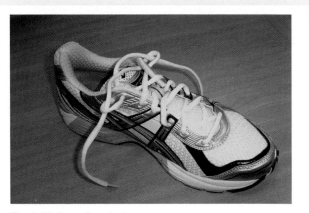

Fig. 1.11 Rear-foot lacing

HOW LONG SHOULD SHOES LAST?

This will depend on your weight, running style, the surface you run on and the amount of training that you do. As a rule of thumb, you should be looking to change every 805km (500 miles), but this will vary if you are a heavy or uneven runner. The best way to check is to look at the spongy layer that sits between your foot and the sole of your trainer. This is the mid-sole and acts as a shock absorber. With use, it gradually becomes more compacted and therefore less able to absorb shock. You can see fatigue lines in the mid-sole which is a sign that you need a new pair.

Listening to your body is also a way to assess the ongoing ability of your trainers to absorb shock. If you start to get new aches and pains in your ankles, knees or hips after running, look at your shoes for signs of fatigue.

Looking after your trainers will also affect how long they last. Don't wash them in the washing machine or dry them on a hot radiator as this will damage the shape of the shoe and affect the function of the mid-sole. Letting trainers dry out slowly will prolong their lifespan; many runners have two or three pairs to allow for this, but it's not essential. All trainers have a shelf life and should be replaced every year anyway.

TWO IS BETTER THAN ONE!

You will get more mileage from your trainers if you alternate between two pairs. You may also find that you are able to haggle a bit of a discount if you buy two pairs at the same time.

ORTHOTICS

Orthotics (see fig. 1.12) are inserts for trainers and shoes that support the muscles, tendons and bones of the feet. When appropriately prescribed, orthotics can decrease pain not only in the foot, but also in other parts of the body such as the knee, hip and lower back. Running can result in a great deal of movement and pressure on the foot. Slight muscle imbalances in the foot that are not usually a problem in day-to-day life may make you more vulnerable to injury when placed under the extra stress of running. Orthotics can help to reduce this stress and fatigue.

Orthotics take various forms, but all have the goal of improving foot function and reducing stress forces that can cause foot deformity and pain. Orthotics can be made in several ways, but most podiatrists make a plaster mould of the patient's foot and send it to a laboratory with a prescription. This allows an orthotic to be made especially for your individual foot to meet your specific needs. Alternatively, you can buy them off the shelf too, but I would recommend seeing a podiatrist who is experienced in making orthotics for runners. This way you will not waste money on insoles that don't work or you don't need, and you will fully understand what to expect from the device.

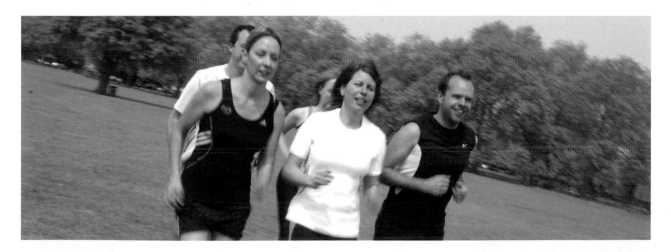

Rigid orthotics

Rigid orthotics are designed to control foot function. These orthotics are mainly designed to control motion in the two major foot joints that lie directly below the ankle joint.

Semi-rigid orthotics

Semi-rigid orthotics allow for dynamic balance of the foot while running and guide the foot through the movement, allowing the muscles and tendons to perform more efficiently.

Soft orthotics

Soft orthotics help to absorb shock, improve balance and take pressure off uncomfortable or sore spots.

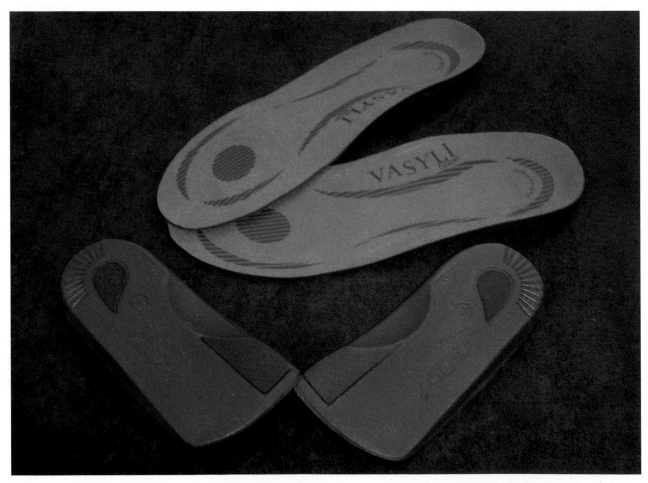

Fig. 1.12: A range of orthotics

YOUR SERVICE HISTORY

Even if you are a regular runner, it's worth stopping every now and again to see where you have come from and to judge what impact this may have on your current running. If you are an inexperienced runner, you definitely need to give some thought to your past so that you can head off any bad habits before they stick.

The questions below are designed to give you a brief 'service history'. After all, you wouldn't think of entering a car in a race or taking it on a long road-trip without knowing what it had been used for in the past. This service history is not designed to give you a full medical check-up – only a professional can do that, so consider a trip to your GP if you are significantly overweight, have any ongoing medical problems or are starting to run later in life.

SERVICE HISTORY	Yes	No
1. Have you run before?		
2. Have you remained free of running injuries in the past?		
3. Are your trainers less than a year old?		
4. Are your trainers specific for your foot type?		
5. Have you run in a different style of trainer before?		
6. Are you training for a specific event?		
7. Have you run this distance before?		
8. If so, did you manage to finish injury free?		
9. Is your training focussed and varied enough for this event?		
10. Are you a member of a running club?		

WEIGHT

To know if you are over- or underweight, you need to work out your body mass index (BMI), which is a measure of your bodyweight in relation to your height. It is not flawless as it doesn't distinguish between muscle and fat, so a muscular person may appear to be overweight when they are not. To work out your BMI, divide your weight (in kilograms) by your height (in metres) squared. For example, if a person weighed 80kg and was 1.70m tall their BMI would be:

80 ÷ (1.7 × 1.7) = 27.68

The 'normal' range for men and women is between 18.5 and 24.9. If your BMI is over 30, try to lose weight before you start running. A healthy diet combined with the gentle walking programme on pages 34–5 is a good place to start and will prevent you putting too much strain on your body, thus avoiding injury and illness. If you have any concerns, you should speak to your doctor who can monitor you as you lose weight.

If your BMI is below 18.5 and you are in good health, don't worry. If you have lost weight recently without dieting or feel unwell, you should see your doctor. If you are a women who has an irregular menstrual cycle or issues with food, again you should see your doctor.

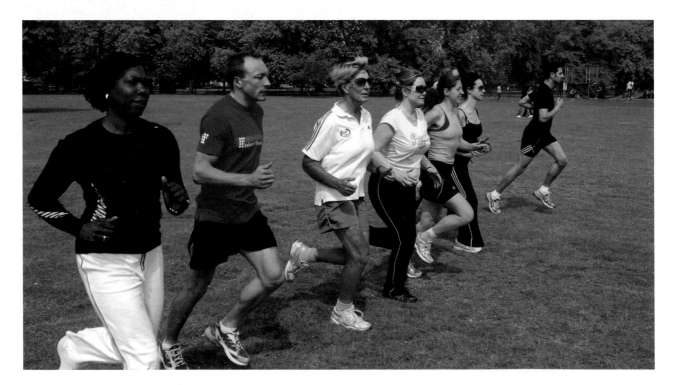

NUTRITION AND HYDRATION

As a runner you are likely to have a healthy, balanced diet already; if you don't, you will soon feel the effects. Imagine driving a car – you would want good quality fuel and you would certainly top up the tank before a journey. Your body is the same – it is just a more complex, highly tuned machine. You may be fit, but it doesn't matter how fit you are if you have insufficient or poor quality fuel – your running will suffer.

Fluid is just as important. Most people function at a level of dehydration and don't drink enough day to day, never mind when they are training. Your body needs 2–2.5 litres of fluid a day to function, and when you are training you will need more. It is important to get the balance right as too much water can be bad for you. There has been a lot of media coverage about the amount of water people should drink at running events due to cases of a condition called hyponatremia (see page 60). The easiest way to keep a check on your hydration levels is to monitor the colour of your urine (see page 61). It should be a pale straw colour; any darker and you're already dehydrated. It is also best to drink isotonic drinks rather than plain water. These drinks have carbohydrate and electrolyte salts mixed in them and will replace any salts lost through sweating.

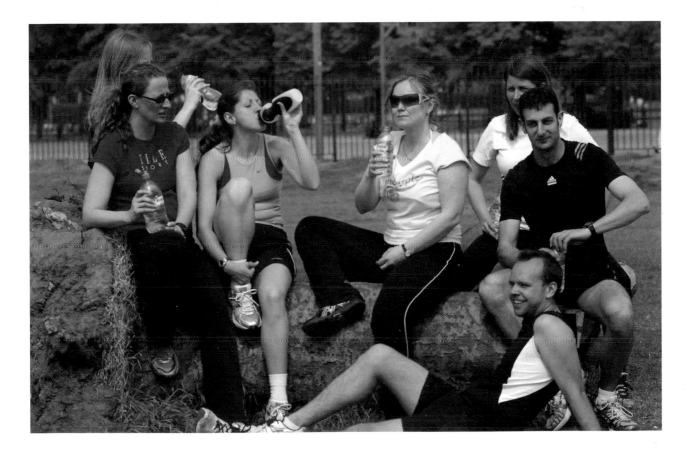

WHERE TO START?

This section is intended to help those who are new to running, and those who answered 'no' frequently in their MOT. I'm not going to suggest detailed training programmes – there are plenty of books out there on this subject. However, many new runners have enjoyed considerable success when following this 'get you started' routine.

Regular exercise can help protect you from heart disease, stroke, high blood pressure, obesity, back pain and osteoporosis, and it can improve your mood and help you manage stress more effectively. For the greatest overall benefits, it is recommended that you do 20–30 minutes of aerobic activity three or more times a week and some type of muscle-strengthening activity, as well as stretching, twice a week. If you are unable to do this, you can gain substantial benefits by accumulating 30 minutes or more of moderate intensity physical activity a day, at least five times a week.

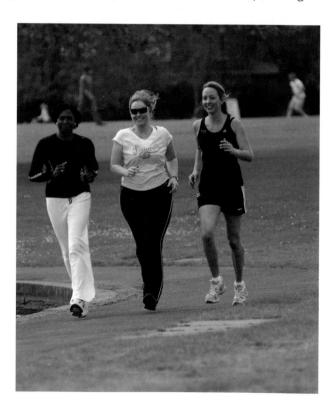

Choose a time of day that suits you, but make sure you have eaten. Don't exercise for at least two hours after eating – this will stop you feeling nauseous. Make sure you sip water during exercise, but don't drink too much – it is more important to drink regularly throughout the day to avoid dehydration rather than too much all in one go.

> **>> FITNESS FACT**
>
> Walk for a few minutes to start your run-walk programme and at the end to cool down. This way you're not ending your session short of breath.

STEADY BEGINNINGS

Brisk walking with a progression to a 'run/walk' programme (where you mix periods of jogging with periods of walking, gradually increasing the duration of the runs and decreasing the frequency of the walk breaks) is a logical place to start. You may prefer to start on a treadmill or cross-trainer at the gym. Both of these prepare the body for running with less impact and also mean you won't be stranded should you feel the need to stop. This allows the body to adapt gradually to the stresses of running, allowing you to avoid injury.

TAKING IT OUTDOORS: WALKING

Walking is not a soft option: you can actually burn more calories walking than running if you vary your walking speed and style. Use the 'little and often' rule and you will see results through a cumulative effect. Using a pedometer helps you to monitor how many steps you take in a day. This means you can make an impact on your fitness without setting foot in a gym. Exercising when and where it suits you and your lifestyle is effective.

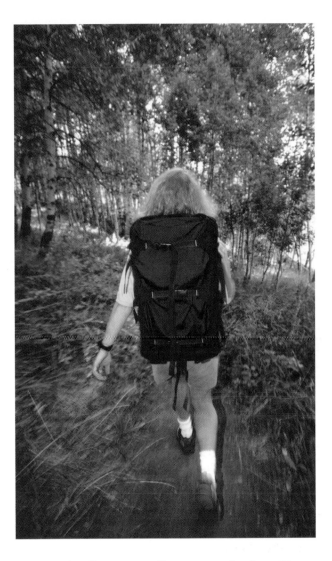

Anyone can walk, but it's an especially good way to ease into exercise if you are unfit or recovering from illness or pregnancy. In the latter case, it may even prove a good way to get your baby off to sleep! It is a low-impact exercise and gets you out in the fresh air, but best of all it is easily accessible and free. By getting off the bus or tube one stop early, or buying your lunch from a shop further away from work, you will walk more and get fitter without really noticing.

Try to maintain a good posture from head to toe, stride out and keep an even pace. Swinging your arms helps to speed up your pace; as you get fitter, you can progress by holding weights as you walk.

WALK SAFE

It is important that you walk on routes that are safe. This includes walking at times of the day when it is light and when places are busy and not secluded if you plan to walk on your own. You can even leave a note at home with the time you left for your walk, where you are going and when you are due back. Take your mobile phone with you so you are always in contact.

BEGINNER'S ROUTINE

This simple routine – I don't like to call it a programme as it is not intended to be that regimented – will build up visible pace and stamina in only a few weeks. Give it a go and you'll be running before you know it.

Weeks 1–2

Start by walking every day. This may be as simple as walking to the train, getting off the bus one stop early or walking to buy your lunch. Taking the stairs instead of the lift also counts as walking and may be possible more than once a day.

Weeks 3–4

The purpose of the first two weeks was to add some walking into your routine without taking up additional time. Now, think about adding an extra 15-minute walk into each day. This may be part of your route to work, a walk to the shops or a walk to a friend's home for coffee. If you are post-natal you could add a walk with your baby to help get them off to sleep.

Weeks 5–6

Increase your daily walking time to 20 minutes in week 5 and 30 minutes in week 6. You can use this time to switch off and have time to yourself or, if you prefer, make phone calls and catch up with all those friends you never get round to calling back. Better still, ask a friend to walk with you and catch up on gossip while you walk.

Weeks 7–8

Now you have an established routine of daily walking it's time to speed things up a little. Introduce swinging your arms and focus on striding out as you walk. See how much further you can walk once you increase your pace. A pedometer will help you to monitor your distance, or alternatively simply use a route you have walked previously in 30 minutes and aim to walk beyond the original finish point.

Weeks 9–10

By now, you should be noticing changes in your fitness – and your waistline! You are ready to progress, and introducing uphill and downhill walking is a great way to improve your cardiovascular fitness. Find a hill either in a park or a street, and walk up it without stopping. Use the walk back down as a recovery to get your breath back; you will still be working your muscles, just in a different way. You can make this a 15-minute part of your workout, as walking to and from the hill is a good warm-up and cool-down.

Weeks 11–12

Another way to progress is to walk while holding weights. These don't have to cost money; they could be two tins of beans. Walk your regular routes and focus on your pace and arm swing. To make sure your grip remains strong, secure the weights to your hands or wrists with string or loops of elastic. For a mixed workout over the week, vary your programme each day: one day with weights, one day with hills and one day on the flat. Keep smiling and walk your way to fitness.

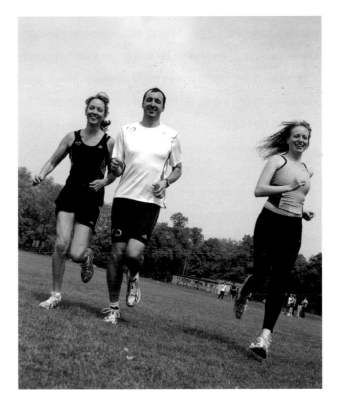

Remember, exercise doesn't have to hurt. Physical pain can be avoided if you exercise within your ability. However, the irritation of changing your routine and becoming disciplined with a commitment to exercise can hurt at first. You should expect muscular aches – this is normal after exercise – but actual pain can be avoided.

Intervals

This is a session that intersperses fast running efforts with periods of recovery. The speed and the length of recovery can be variable depending on what you want to achieve, and your fitness level. It is important not to run the sets too fast – it is not sprint training. Aim to run each repeat at the same pace; if the earlier sets were faster than the final few, this means you started out too fast.

Hills training

This session will usually involve repeats on a particular hill or a specific gradient on a treadmill. You can include hills on any run so the route is undulating, but this is different from a pure hills session. You will increase your cardiovascular fitness as well as developing strength in your legs.

Fartlek

Fartlek training, which originated in Scandinavia, is similar to interval training. Fartlek means speed play, and involves running in fast, hard bursts as and when you feel up to it during a steady run. These sessions help to increase your pace over a steady run without having to increase the distance. It's a great way to increase your pace generally or re-introduce speed work to your sessions after injury or illness.

Tempo/threshold runs

These are fast sessions running at a pace that won't allow you to keep chatting! They usually last between 20 and 30 minutes and bring you to the brink of your lactate/anaerobic threshold. Working at this intensity allows your body to raise the lactate threshold, which means you will be able to run for longer as your body becomes more efficient at removing lactic acid from the muscle. The benefits are physiological, in that you will be able to produce energy at a higher intensity but you will also notice your pace increase.

Strength and conditioning exercises

It is important to build strength in your muscles to prevent injury. Running is excellent for cardiovascular fitness, but weight training and conditioning to maintain and strengthen muscles will minimise the repetitive effects of running, and facilitate your body's ability to maintain dynamic biomechanics in the lower limb.

Cross-training

It is important to give your body a rest from the repetitive movement and impact of running. Cross-training allows you to train while giving your running muscles a break. Cross-training includes cycling, swimming, the cross-trainer machine and gym work.

Dynamic and passive stretching

Stretching is often overlooked. Stretches should be performed to maintain functional muscle length and help prevent muscle imbalances. The latest research suggests that passive stretching prior to running is not helpful, but that stretching after a run is effective. Dynamic stretching is a great way to improve the flexibility of muscles prior to and after running, and is an effective conditioning drill when cross-training.

Massage

Intense training can cause increases in muscle tone, which is often felt as tightness or a knot. If this is allowed to remain it can impair the delivery of oxygen and nutrients to the muscle. This can cause fatigue in the legs, affecting your training, and can also affect the removal of metabolites and other waste products of exercise, effectively slowing recovery. Muscle imbalances can also develop if tightness is allowed to persist, and this can also lead to injury. Massage is an important part of maintaining the condition of your muscles when you are training, and is more than just a luxury.

Running with water/dog

Carrying water on a long run is essential, but make sure it is a small bottle or carried in a running belt. This will ensure your arm swing and running technique is not affected. Running with your dog on the lead will have a similar effect – if your dog is well-trained, have him/her run alongside you.

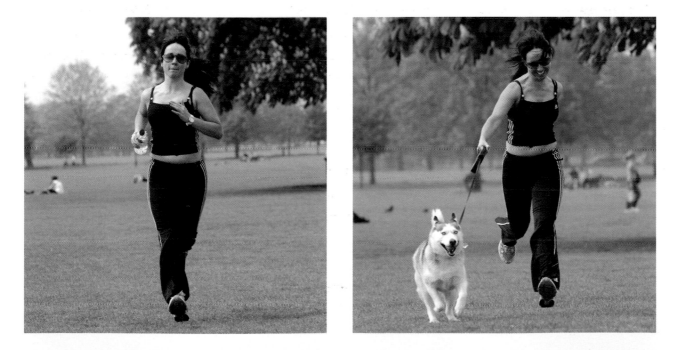

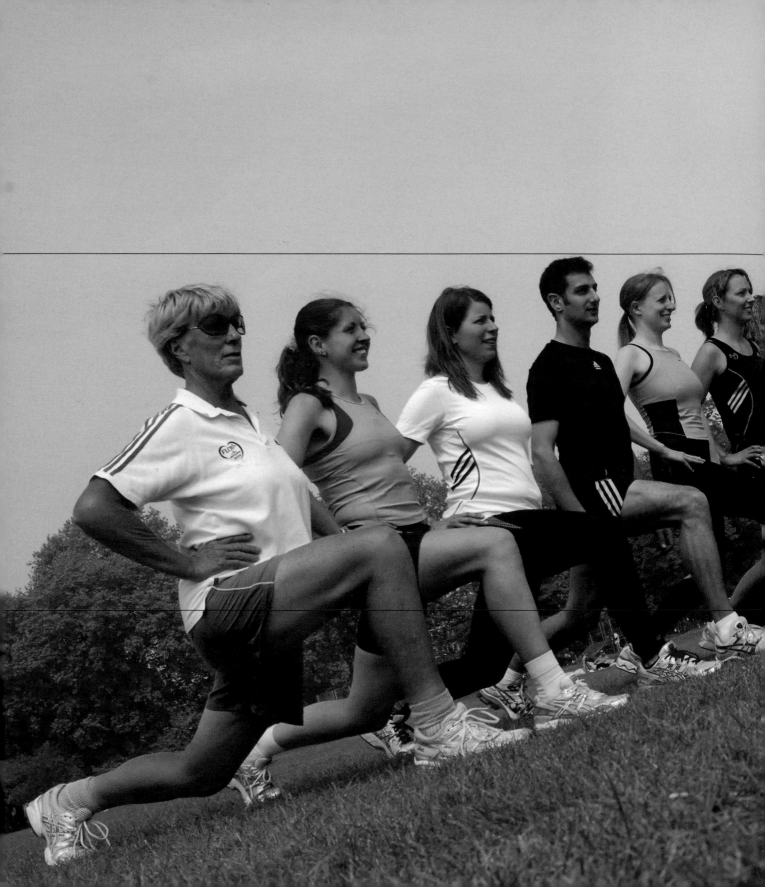

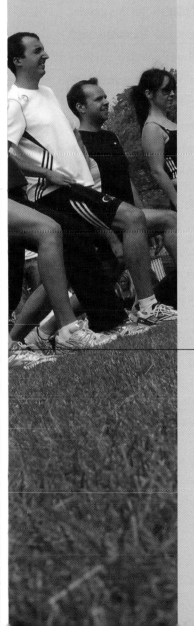

2

THE USUAL SUSPECTS

In this chapter I will show you how to identify injuries and then to answer the questions you should be asking yourself. This will help you to correctly manage yourself immediately after the injury. I will then guide you through further considerations to assist the healing process, explaining what you have done and what you need to do to get back into your trainers and out running towards your goal. Just follow the easy-to-use traffic light system, which shows what you can do to treat yourself and helps you to know when you need to seek professional advice and treatment.

CONTENTS

HOW CAN I MAKE IT BETTER?

You will see that each injury has a 'traffic light' system of treatment. This is designed to make it easy for you to treat your injury and advises when you should get straight to a specialist.

MEET THE SPECIALISTS

You will notice that I have recommended that you seek the help of various specialists for some of the injuries. It is unlikely that you will need the services of all these professionals during your running days, but it doesn't hurt to know who they are.

The physiotherapist

Physiotherapy sees full and functional movement at the heart of what it means to be healthy. Working with a physiotherapist will allow you to develop, maintain and restore movement and function after injury. A physiotherapist will also identify and maximise your movement potential within the areas of health promotion and injury prevention, alongside treatment and rehabilitation.

As a runner you can benefit greatly from a physiotherapist's assessment, diagnostic skills and subsequent intervention strategies to get you pain free, back from injury and prevent further training issues and movement dysfunctions.

TREATMENT TRAFFIC LIGHT

Self-treatment

This is the self-treatment you can start immediately to manage your injury and prevent it becoming worse.

Seek medical advice

You may need assessment and treatments. A physiotherapist or healthcare professional will be able to advise you on how to manage your injury.

Seek medical attention

Things are serious and you need assessment to rule out complications and to take advice on the best way to manage this injury. Your physio may also arrange this for you.

The osteopath and chiropractor

Osteopathy and chiropractics are both branches of complementary medicine that not only take into account your physical symptoms, but also your lifestyle, attitudes and current health. The underlying philosophy is that the body has a natural tendency to heal itself, but this can be disrupted by imbalances in the musculoskeletal system. An osteopath investigates a patient's symptoms using many of the diagnostic procedures from conventional medicine. The patient is assessed on a mechanical, functional and postural basis. Manual methods of treatment appropriate to the individual patient are then applied.

The podiatrist

Podiatry is the field of healthcare devoted to the study and treatment of disorders of the foot and ankle and the function of the lower extremity. Podiatrists work closely with physiotherapists in the management and prevention of running injuries and are the experts in biomechanical assessment. They will prescribe custom-made orthotics if you require help to control the foot position when running. This can have a great impact on injury prevention and muscle imbalance issues.

The chiropodist

Chiropody treatment for the runner is essential. Treatments include reducing hard skin, treatment to corns and calluses, laser treatment for heel pain and verrucae and nail surgery. Podiatry and chiropody are similar professions, with the main difference being the area of speciality.

The pharmacist

Your high street pharmacist is the best person to advise you on which medications can help you without a prescription and what to have in your first aid kit. If you run regularly, you will already know the benefits of having the basics at hand. You should also go to the pharmacist to get stocks of plasters, blister care products and treatment for fungal infections and athlete's foot. Use the same pharmacist for all of your prescription and non-prescription drugs as they can then monitor what you take and warn if there any any unwanted interactions between different drugs.

The sports physician

A referral to a sports physician is required when self-management and physiotherapy have not helped after 4–6 weeks. Your physiotherapist or GP will refer you so that further assessment and investigations can be made.

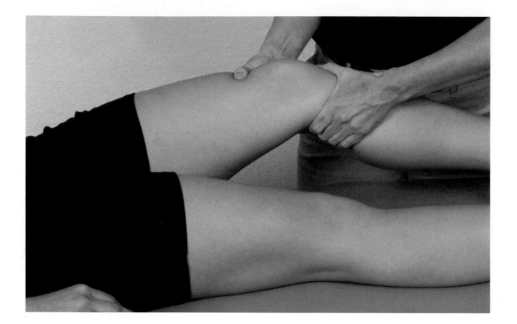

>> **FITNESS FACT**

Learn to read and listen to your body's language. Especially when you have aches and pains, feel fatigued, hungry or thirsty.

The sports masseuse

A good masseuse is invaluable and will work closely with your physiotherapist to manage your sporting fitness. For many, a massage is a luxury, but as a runner it is essential to keep your legs in shape after heavy training sessions. It is also a great way to address muscle imbalances alongside your physiotherapy treatment or stretch programme.

NHS Direct

This is a useful service that can offer advice if you are concerned but unable to see your physiotherapist or GP. NHS Direct can help you make a decision on the most appropriate management for your injury and advise you on who you should see if things become worse. Check out www.nhsdirect.nhs.uk.

>> **FITNESS FACT**

After a race allow one day recovery for every mile run. This will allow your body to repair and stay injury free when you start to run again.

A&E

Your local hospital A&E department is for accidents and emergencies only. You may be in a lot of pain, but most sports injuries are not an emergency and do not require A&E services. You will only have a very long wait as others are seen before you. If your hospital has a minor injuries unit, that will be a more appropriate location for treatment and advice.

The sports dietician

Most people would benefit from dietary advice but, as a runner, it is as easy to overeat as it is to undereat. Simple advice can have a major impact on your training, allowing you to eat foods specific to the session you have on a certain day or ensuring that vitamin and mineral intake is maintained so increases in training do not impact heavily on your health.

> **>> FITNESS FACT**
>
> Change your diet for life not just the race. The benefit to you will be much greater and will affect more than just performance.

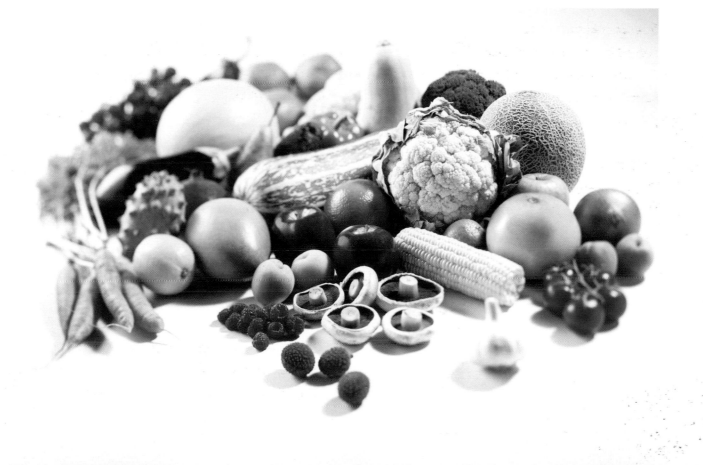

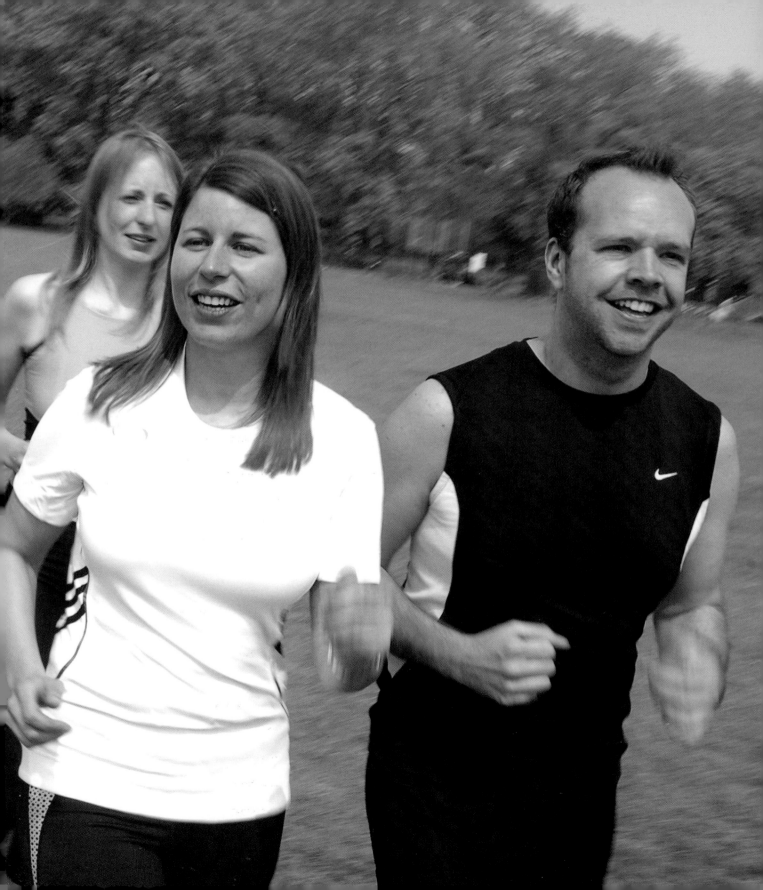

HEAD AND TRUNK

Running injuries here are slightly different from injuries elsewhere. The impact on the muscles and how they are used relates more to your everyday posture and your running posture. Aspects of your lifestyle have a direct impact on the head and trunk, especially dehydration, stress and postural pain. In this section you will find suggestions to help you to manage and prevent these symptoms.

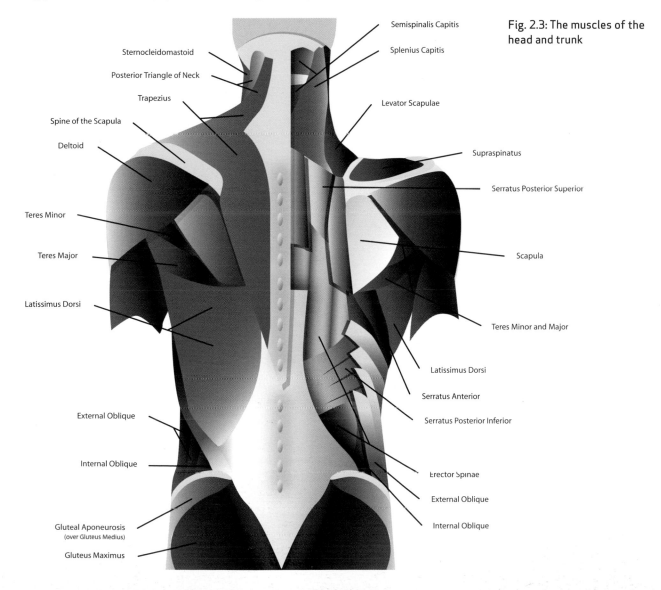

Fig. 2.3: The muscles of the head and trunk

Semispinalis Capitis
Splenius Capitis
Sternocleidomastoid
Posterior Triangle of Neck
Trapezius
Levator Scapulae
Spine of the Scapula
Deltoid
Supraspinatus
Serratus Posterior Superior
Teres Minor
Teres Major
Scapula
Latissimus Dorsi
Teres Minor and Major
Latissimus Dorsi
Serratus Anterior
Serratus Posterior Inferior
External Oblique
Internal Oblique
Erector Spinae
External Oblique
Internal Oblique
Gluteal Aponeurosis
(over Gluteus Medius)
Gluteus Maximus

POSTURAL BACK AND NECK PAIN

Muscle or ligament strains and fatigue are the most common cause of postural back pain. Nearly everyone will experience postural back pain at some point in their life, especially these days with the increase in sedentary jobs and hobbies based around computers and computer games. Long commutes in the car or train don't help either.

SYMPTOMS

Aching, spasm, tightness and restricted movement. See below for areas of pain.

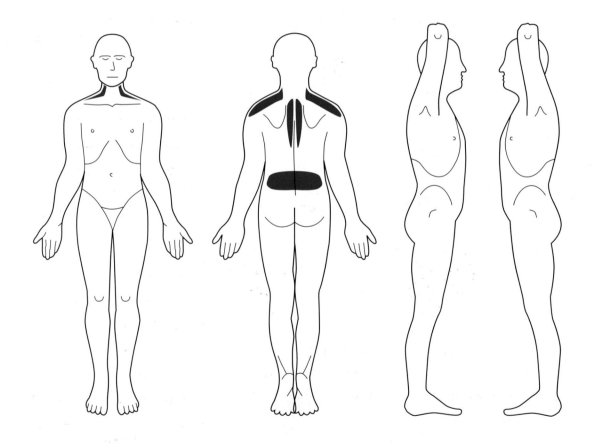

Aggravated by :	Eased by:
Prolonged sitting	Movement
Prolonged standing	Changing position
Driving for over one hour	Stretch breaks

The spinal vertebrae are connected by tough ligaments and muscles that help to maintain the position of the spinal column. These muscles and ligaments work together to provide control and strength for nearly all activities (and 'inactivities'). You still need postural muscle control to sit at your desk and computer game console! I'm often asked, "What is the best spinal posture?" and I have to say it's the next one you move into. Any posture can become painful if you stay in it for too long.

PREDISPOSING FACTORS

- Working long hours
- Driving long distances/commuting
- Carrying heavy bags or laptops
- Poor spinal stability
- Poor strength and conditioning
- Obesity
- Smoking
- Poor lifting technique
- Previous episodes of experiencing low-back pain
- Poor ergonomics at work or in the car
- Hypermobility

If you have persistent problems, you should consider these factors. If you smoke, are overweight or do not perform regular back-strengthening exercises, changing your lifestyle can help you control your symptoms.

TREATMENT TRAFFIC LIGHT

Self-treatment

- Simple stretches
- Changes to your workstation ergonomics (see page 119)
- Getting fit
- Postural awareness
- Get the right laptop bag for your journeys
- Use a laptop stand and external keyboard when out of the office

Seek medical advice

- Acupuncture
- Stretching and strengthening
- Spinal stability training
- Pilates/yoga/Alexander technique/Method Pukitso
- Mobilisation and manipulation
- Massage

Seek medical attention

- Dizziness and blackouts
- Blurred vision
- Ringing in the ears
- Slurred speech
- Progressive weakness in the limbs
- Severe, constant pain that is not relieved by lying down
- Constant pins and needles or numbness in the limbs
- Shortness of breath

STRESS AND ANXIETY

Stress can result from any situation or thought that makes you feel frustrated, angry or anxious. The things that make you feel stressed are not necessarily stressful to someone else. Anxiety is best described as a feeling of apprehension or fear. You may not know or recognise the reason for feeling uneasy, and this can make you feel more distressed.

It has to be said that stress is a normal part of life and, in small amounts, stress is good. You can use it to motivate you and help you to be more productive or train harder. However, too much stress, or a strong response to stress, is not so good for you. It can lead to you feeling generally unwell, as well as leading to physical or psychological illness like infection, heart disease or depression. Persistent and unrelenting stress often leads to anxiety and other unhealthy behaviours like overeating, binge drinking or taking drugs. Recognising stress and anxiety and how you respond to it is very important.

SYMPTOMS

Anxiety is often accompanied by physical symptoms, such as:

- Twitching or trembling
- Muscle tension headaches
- Sweating
- Dry mouth and difficulty swallowing
- Abdominal pain
- Dizziness
- Rapid or irregular heart rate
- Rapid breathing
- Diarrhoea or frequent need to urinate
- Fatigue
- Irritability, including loss of temper
- Sleeping difficulties and nightmares
- Decreased concentration
- Sexual problems.

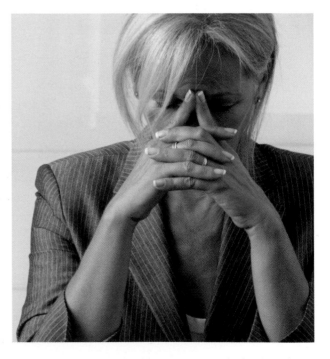

Aggravated by:	Eased by:
Being injured	Insight to the problem
Work	Coping strategies
Family	Time out
Moving house	Professional help
Relationships	Goal setting

PREDISPOSING FACTORS

- Certain drugs, both recreational and medicinal (bronchodilators for asthma, tricyclic antidepressants, cocaine, amphetamines, diet pills, ADHD medications and thyroid medications)
- High caffeine intake
- Smoking/alcohol abuse
- Poor diet
- Low levels of Vitamin B12
- Performance anxiety related to specific situations, like starting a race you have trained hard for or making a presentation in public
- Post-traumatic stress disorder (PTSD), which can develop after a traumatic event like terrorism, physical or sexual assault or a natural disaster

The most effective solution is to find and address the source of your stress or anxiety. This is not always easy or possible and you may need help to do so. A first step is to make a list of what you think might be making you feel anxious or stressed:

- What do you worry about most?
- Is something constantly on your mind?
- Does anything in particular make you sad or depressed?

Then, find someone you trust (friend, family member, priest, healthcare professional) who will listen to you. Often, just talking to a friend is all that is needed to relieve anxiety. It is also important to find healthy ways to cope with and manage your stress.

Your doctor can help you determine if your anxiety would be best evaluated and treated by a mental healthcare professional.

TREATMENT TRAFFIC LIGHT

Self-treatment

- Eat a well-balanced, healthy diet
- Get enough sleep
- Exercise regularly, but don't overtrain
- Limit caffeine and alcohol intake
- Don't use nicotine, cocaine or other recreational drugs
- Learn and practise relaxation techniques, like guided imagery or progressive muscle relaxation
- Yoga, tai chi, or meditation
- Make sure you balance fun activities with responsibilities
- Spend time with friends

Seek medical advice

- Acupuncture
- Massage
- Hypnotherapy

Seek medical attention

- Unable to function properly
- Do not know the cause of anxiety
- Sudden feeling of panic
- Uncontrollable fear, for example, of becoming unwell if outside
- Repeating an action, like constantly washing hands
- Intolerance to heat; weight loss, despite a good appetite; a lump/swelling in the front of your neck; protruding eyes. (The thyroid may be overactive.)
- Anxiety is made worse by the memory of a traumatic event
- Tried self-care for several weeks without success, or feel that any anxiety will not resolve without professional help

HYPONATREMIA

This is a condition to avoid at all costs. As you compete in more races, it is important to monitor your hydration during both training and racing. Hyponatremia is a condition also known as 'water intoxication'. It is the opposite of dehydration and is not an unusual problem – and you can develop it in a few hours.

Most people when running think they will sweat too much and so drink a lot of water before and during a race. If you consume large amounts of water over the course of a day, blood plasma (the liquid part of blood) increases and dilutes the salt content of the blood. At the same time, your body loses salt by sweating. This results in a decreased amount of electrolytes available to your body. Over time, this will interfere with brain, heart and muscle function. These electrolytes are essential in maintaining the normal electro-chemical operation of your body and nervous system.

The imbalance of water to salt is caused by one of three conditions:

1. Hypovolemic hyponatremia: water and sodium are both lost from the body, but the sodium loss is greater.

2. Hypervolemic hyponatremia: both sodium and water content in the body increase, but the water gain is greater.

3. Euvolemic hyponatremia: there is an increase in total body water, but the sodium content remains constant.

Watch out for the following symptoms: apathy, confusion, nausea and fatigue. You can prevent them by:

- making sure you are sufficiently hydrated.
- never reaching the point of feeling thirsty.
- ensuring your urine is always as pale as possible; if it is dark; you are already dehydrated (see Fig. 2.3 opposite).
- sipping at water throughout the day rather than gulping it down.

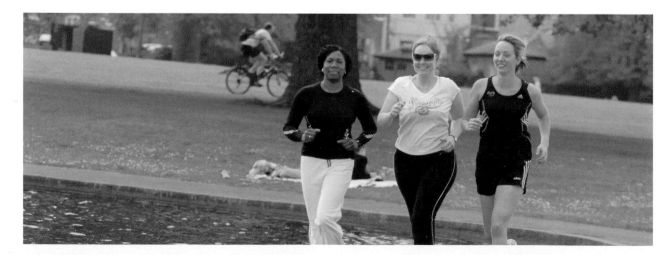

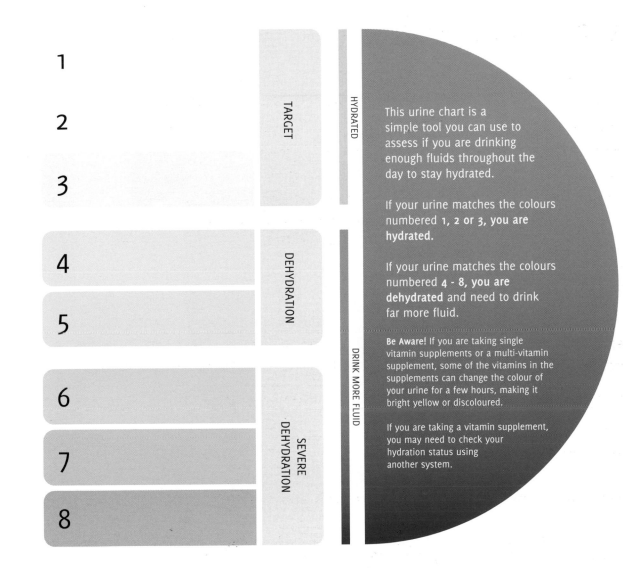

TARGET

DEHYDRATION

SEVERE DEHYDRATION

HYDRATED

DRINK MORE FLUID

This urine chart is a simple tool you can use to assess if you are drinking enough fluids throughout the day to stay hydrated.

If your urine matches the colours numbered 1, 2 or 3, you are **hydrated.**

If your urine matches the colours numbered **4 - 8, you are dehydrated** and need to drink far more fluid.

Be Aware! If you are taking single vitamin supplements or a multi-vitamin supplement, some of the vitamins in the supplements can change the colour of your urine for a few hours, making it bright yellow or discoloured.

If you are taking a vitamin supplement, you may need to check your hydration status using another system.

Fig. 2.4 Hydration chart showing colour of urine when hydrated/dehydrated.

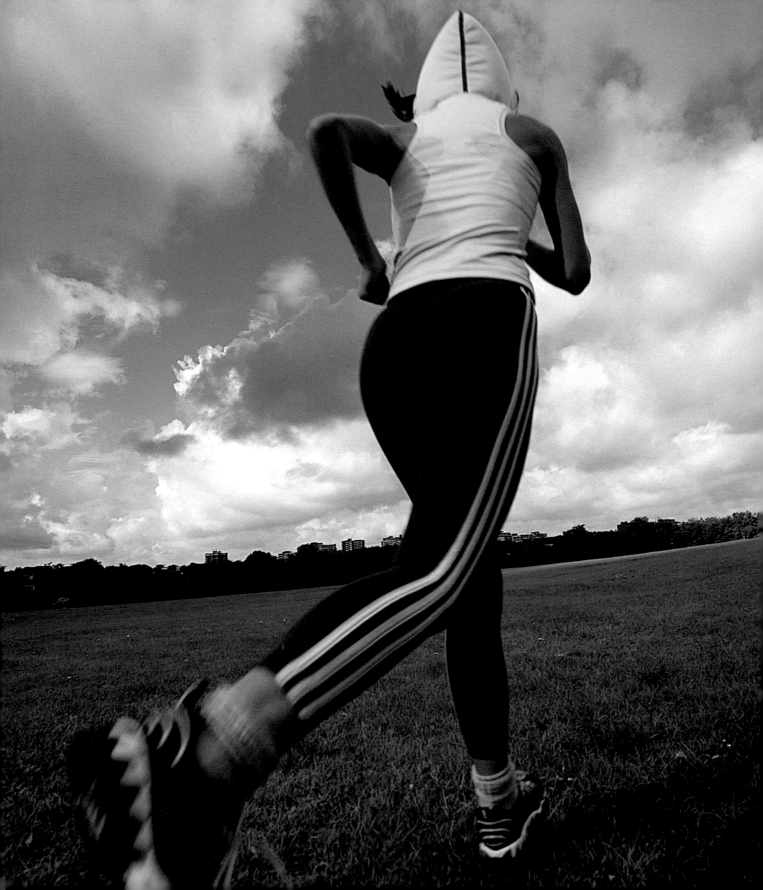

LOWER BACK, HIPS AND THIGHS

This part of the body is the power house and core upon which the body builds its stability and strength. The majority of injuries are muscular in origin but, if not treated properly, can develop into bigger problems that may affect the nerves and joints of the spine, hips and knees. It is important that you have the strength and flexibility in this area to prevent injury. Reading through this section will help you to identify symptoms that you may have, then show you the exercise that will get you back to running if you are currently injured, and keep you running by improving your strength if you recognise areas of weakness in yourself.

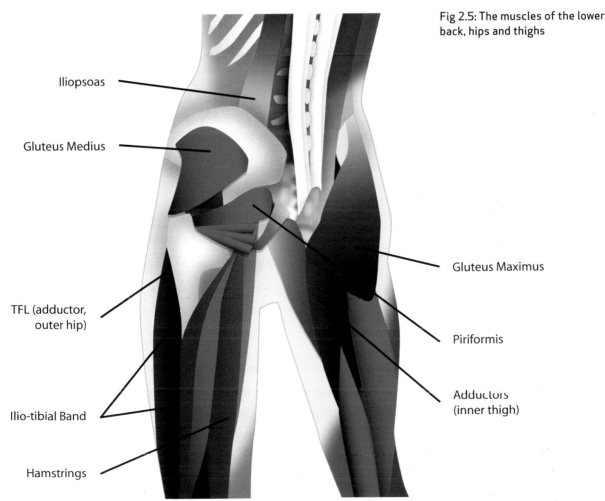

Fig 2.5: The muscles of the lower back, hips and thighs

Iliopsoas

Gluteus Medius

Gluteus Maximus

TFL (adductor, outer hip)

Piriformis

Adductors (inner thigh)

Ilio-tibial Band

Hamstrings

PIRIFORMIS SYNDROME

The piriformis muscle is a small muscle that runs from the sacrum (base of the spine) to the outer hip bone. If the piriformis becomes tight or cramps, it can put pressure on the sciatic nerve, which passes underneath the muscle. You may be one of the 15 per cent of people whose piriformis is split into two, with the nerve passing between the two muscle bellies. Buttock pain is a common symptom, but piriformis syndrome is also a common cause of sciatica (leg pain).

SYMPTOMS

See below for areas of pain.

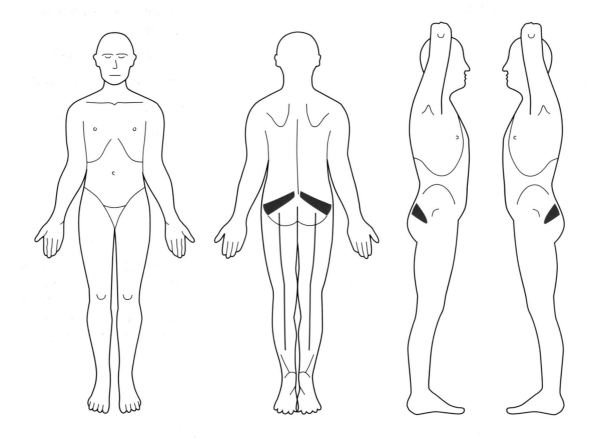

Aggravated by :	Eased by:
Sitting	Rest
Activity	Activity
Pressure to the area	Stretching

Shortening of the muscle and compression of the nerve is the most common cause of piriformis syndrome, but overuse of the glutes and other muscles in the hip can also cause muscle spasm in the piriformis.

PREDISPOSING FACTORS

- Poor biomechanics
- Weak glutes
- Poor flexibility
- Poor running technique
- Old or the wrong trainers
- Being female: 6:1 ratio

TREATMENT TRAFFIC LIGHT

Self-treatment

- Stretching
- Strengthening
- Simple analgesia
- Don't overtrain

Seek advice

- Wearing the right trainers for your foot type
- Biomechanical assessment
- Gait analysis of your running style
- Acupuncture
- Massage

Seek medical attention

- If pain persists or becomes worse with stretching, you should see your physiotherapist to ensure that it is not pain that is referred to the buttock and leg from the spine.

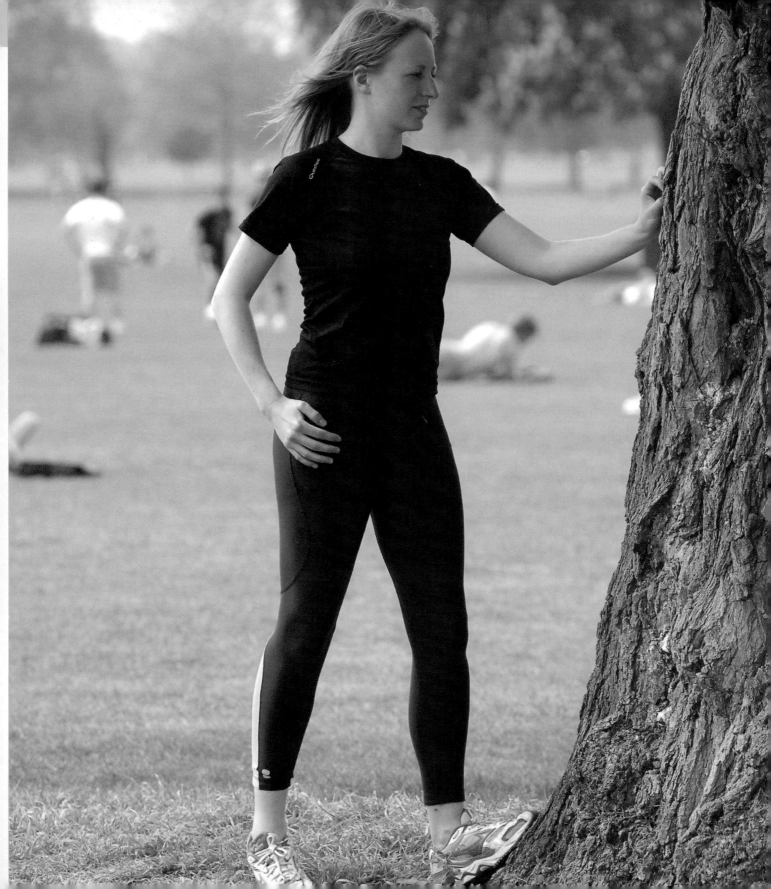

DELAYED-ONSET MUSCLE SORENESS (DOMS)

Delayed-onset muscle soreness after exercise is not uncommon, particularly if you are beginning an exercise programme or changing your training programme. Some muscle soreness may be felt from 12–48 hours following the activity; you may also experience muscle stiffness, fatigue and weakness. Be assured, this is a normal response as your muscles adapt to the new exercise and stresses. Over time, this adaptation leads to greater muscle strength and endurance and the same training session will no longer result in soreness. DOMS is generally worst within the first 2 days following the activity and subsides over the next few days.

PREVENTING DOMS

- Warm up thoroughly before activity and cool down completely afterwards. Perform easy stretching after exercise.
- Start a new training programme gradually and build up duration and intensity over time.
- When lifting weight, start with light weights and high reps (10–12) and gradually increase the amount you lift over several weeks.
- Avoid making sudden changes in the distances you run.
- Avoid making sudden changes in the speed you run.

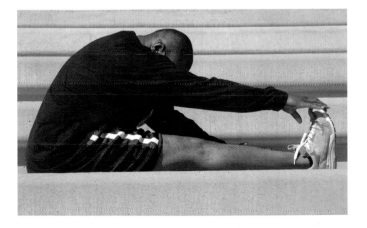

>> **FITNESS FACT**

Take an extra rest before and after a race. The longer the race, the longer you will need to prepare and recover.

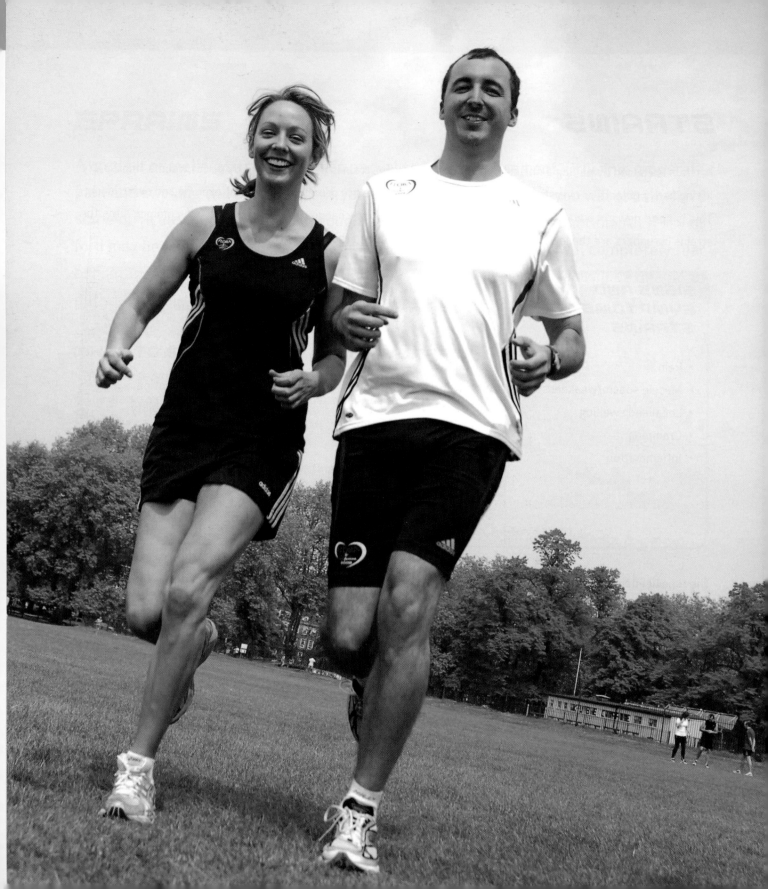

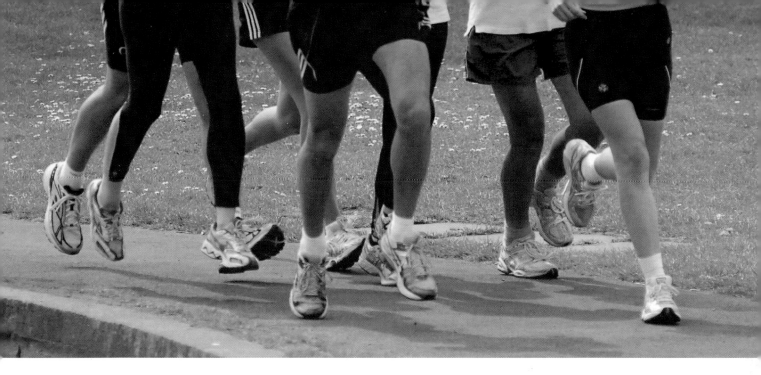

KNEES AND SHINS

Non-runners seem to be obsessed about the knees of runners – there seems to be a fixation with the idea that we are literally running our knees into the ground with every step we take! In truth, knee injuries are not inevitable and though common, are easily treated if properly managed and, even better news, knee pain need not stop you from running. The knee is one of the most complex joints in the body and pain usually results from overuse, poor form during physical activity, or inadequate stretching. Simple causes of knee pain often clear up on their own or with self-management. Being overweight can put you at greater risk of knee problems.

There are many things that can be injured around the knee joint and the exact location of the pain can help identify the structure involved. Pain on the front of the knee can be due to bursitis, tendonitis, arthritis or chondromalacia; pain on the sides of the knee is commonly related to injuries to the collateral ligaments, arthritis or tears to the meniscae; and pain in the back of the knee can be caused by arthritis, meniscal tears or a Baker's cyst, which is an accumulation of joint fluid (synovial fluid) that forms behind the knee.

Overall knee pain can be due to all of the above or instability. Instability, locking, clicking or giving way are other common symptoms. These symptoms are usually associated with damage to the meniscus or structural ligaments after a twisting injury or a history of injuries in the joint.

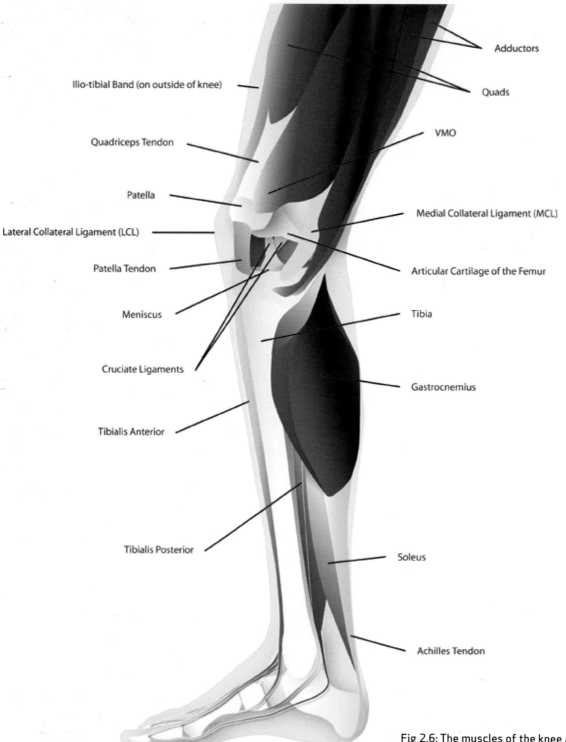

Adductors

Quads

VMO

Ilio-tibial Band (on outside of knee)

Quadriceps Tendon

Patella

Lateral Collateral Ligament (LCL)

Patella Tendon

Meniscus

Cruciate Ligaments

Tibialis Anterior

Tibialis Posterior

Medial Collateral Ligament (MCL)

Articular Cartilage of the Femur

Tibia

Gastrocnemius

Soleus

Achilles Tendon

Fig 2.6: The muscles of the knee and shin

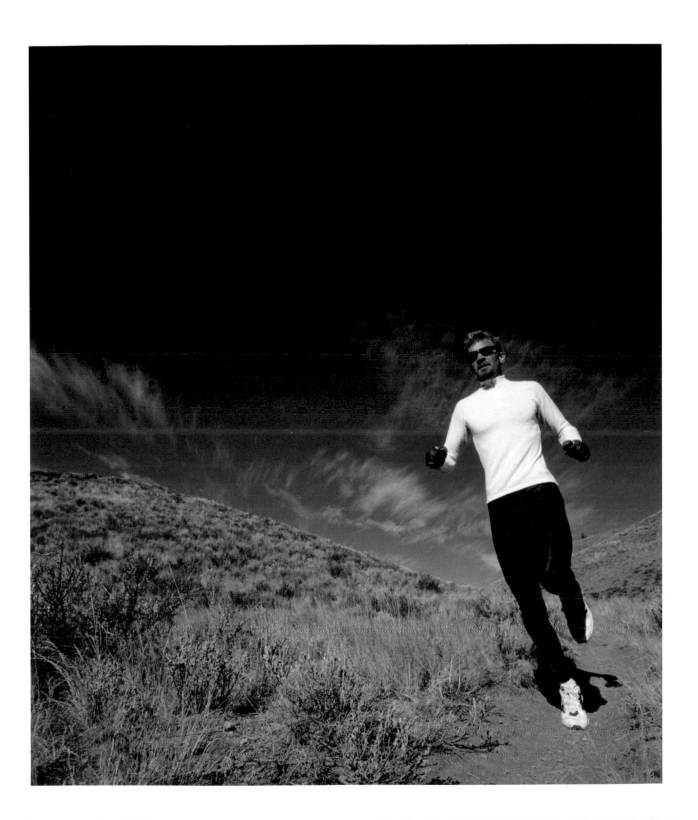

PATELLOFEMORAL PAIN SYNDROME

The knee is one of the most complex joints in the human body and is prone to a variety of sports-related injuries. One of the more common is patellofemoral pain syndrome. While the exact cause of patellofemoral pain isn't known, it is likely to have something to do with the way the patella tracks along the groove of the femur. The patella can move up and down and from side to side in the groove, as well as tilt and rotate. The patella depends upon muscle strength and balance to prevent overuse and incorrect tracking. If the patella is maltracking, it can cause inflammation that will result in pain.

SYMPTOMS

Pain under and around the knee cap. See below for areas of pain.

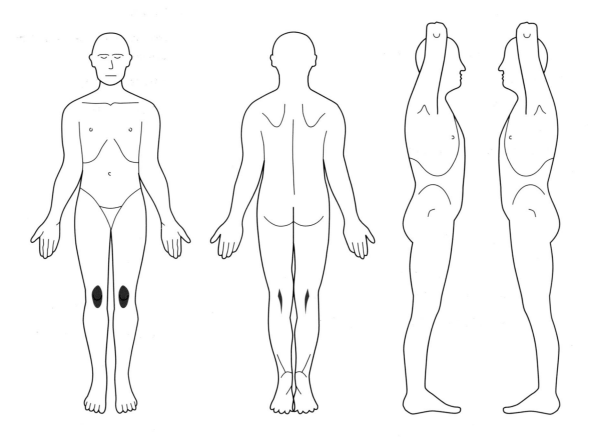

Aggravated by:	Eased by:
Activity	Rest
Walking downstairs	Ice
Long periods of inactivity	Anti-inflammatories
Squatting	

Despite all the things that may cause the pain, there are specific things you can do to combat patellofemoral pain. Rest is one of the first lines of defence. Turn to non-impact exercise, such as swimming or the cross-trainer, to keep your fitness level while allowing your pain to settle. A physiotherapist is the best person to teach you a specific treatment plan. Depending upon the results of your assessment, you will need to add strengthening and stretching exercises to your routine.

PREDISPOSING FACTORS

- Muscle imbalances
- Worn-out or the wrong style shoes
- Tight muscles in the thigh and hip
- Tracking problems due to patella position
- Overtraining

PATELLOFEMORAL PAIN

Patellofemoral pain can be hard to treat, and treatment may take a considerable amount of time. I would always advise an assessment with a physiotherapist in order to be sure of your diagnosis.

TREATMENT TRAFFIC LIGHT

Self-treatment

- Ice the knees after exercise
- Rest from running and maintain fitness with cross-training
- Strengthening exercises for the quadriceps and gluteals
- Stretches
- Correct footwear

Seek medical advice

- Orthotics after assessment from a podiatrist
- Soft-tissue massage
- Taping the patella

Seek medical attention

- Ease into an exercise routine
- Learn specific quadriceps strength exercises
- Wear appropriate footwear
- Rest at any signs of overuse

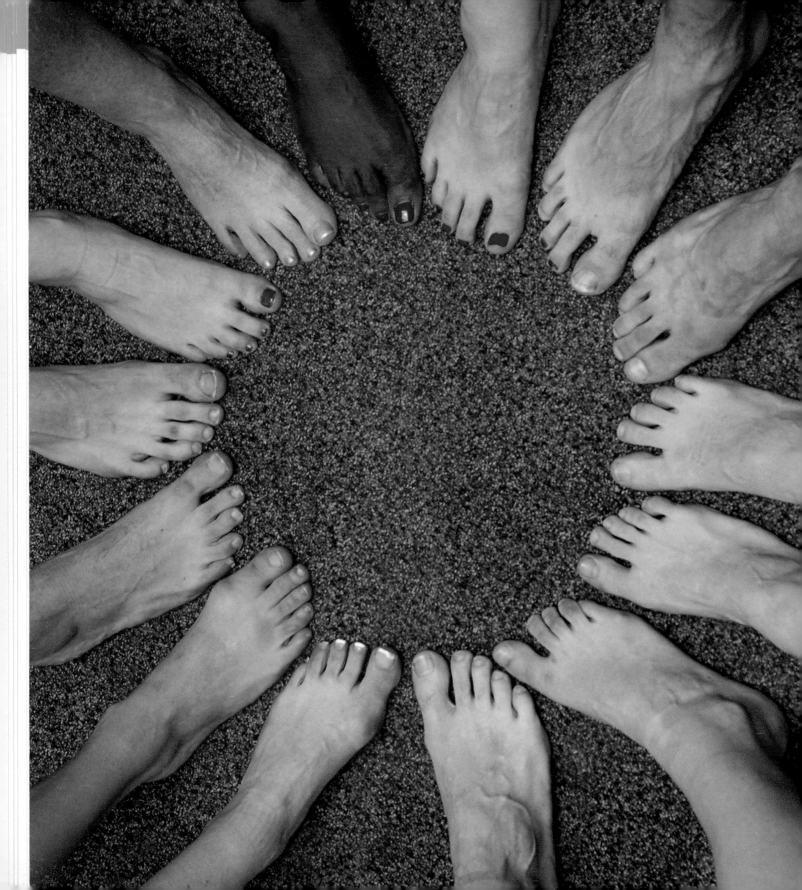

FEET AND ANKLES

The feet and ankles could be described as the most important part of a runner's body, which is why they must be looked after and encased in the best trainers for your foot type. This is the part of the body that makes direct contact with the ground and transmits those forces up through the leg. Strength and posture in the feet must be matched by the strength and position of the hip to protect the knee from injury and excessive rotational forces through the leg. The way in which the foot strikes the ground and pushes off again is open to change, and making sure that your running technique is as good as it can be is essential for injury prevention not only in this area but through the leg and spine too.

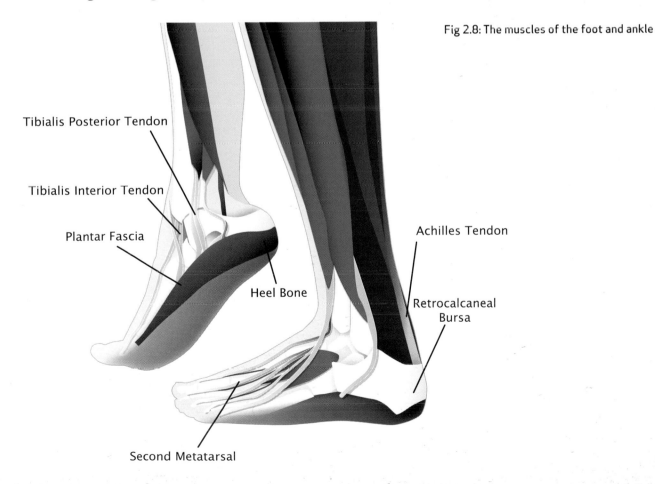

Fig 2.8: The muscles of the foot and ankle

Tibialis Posterior Tendon

Tibialis Interior Tendon

Plantar Fascia

Heel Bone

Achilles Tendon

Retrocalcaneal Bursa

Second Metatarsal

PLANTAR FASCIITIS

Plantar fasciitis is considered a chronic injury and is the most common cause of pain at the arch of the foot and heel. This is because it develops over time rather than having a sudden cause. It is common in runners due to the repetitive push-off movement of the toes. The plantar fascia (a broad, ligament-like structure extending from the heel bone to the base of the toes) provides support for the medial longitudinal arch of the foot and is stretched as the arch flattens slightly to absorb the impact each time the heel strikes the ground. The fascia is not very flexible and repetitive stretching from impact can result in small tears.

SYMPTOMS

See below for areas of pain.

Plantar Fasciitis

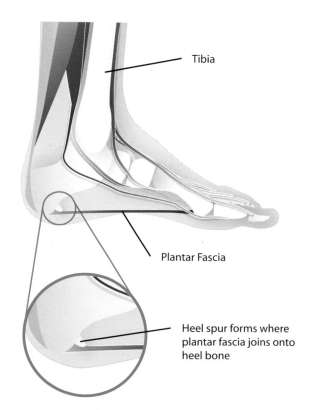

Tibia

Plantar Fascia

Heel spur forms where plantar fascia joins onto heel bone

Fig 2.9: Plantar fasciitis and heel spurs

Heel pain during the first steps of the morning is a classic sign. This pain is the result of the foot resting in plantar flexion (toes pointed) overnight, allowing the fascia to shorten. When the shortened fascia is stretched when you stand, it is painful. Pain continues when the inflammation becomes chronic and the small tears in the fascia don't heal. A heel spur (see page 102), which gives pain in the centre of the heel, can be a sign of fasciitis, but is not a cause. About half of patients with plantar fasciitis will have heel spurs.

Aggravated by:	Eased by:
First steps in the morning	Activity/use
Beginning activity after a long rest	Ice
Start of a run/exercise	Massage

PREDISPOSING FACTORS

- Flat feet
- High arches
- Excessive pronation
- Obesity or sudden weight gain
- Tight Achilles tendons
- Sudden increase in running intensity, time or distance
- Wearing shoes with poor cushioning or support
- Change in running or walking surface
- Occupation with prolonged standing

TREATMENT TRAFFIC LIGHT

Self-treatment

- Avoid painful activities and barefoot walking on hard surfaces
- Weight loss when appropriate
- Achilles and plantar fascia stretches (see pages 148–159)
- Massage the fascia by rolling your foot over a rolling pin or soup can; freeze a small bottle of water and roll your foot over that to combine massage and ice (see page 152)
- Strengthening exercises

Seek medical advice

- Non-steroidal anti-inflammatory drugs (NSAIDs) can be used for 2–4 weeks in conjunction with other treatments (check with your doctor/pharmacist for specific instructions)
- Taping the heel and arch may also help reduce pain
- Medial longitudinal arch supports can be used if they produce a positive result
- Proper footwear with arch support is recommended

Seek medical attention

- If symptoms do not respond to treatment in 1–2 weeks, things may be more serious. Always consult a physician for a thorough evaluation and diagnosis.

HEEL SPURS

A heel spur is a growth of bone on the bottom of the heel where the muscles and the plantar fascia attach. If heel pain is treated early, heel spurs can be prevented.

SYMPTOMS

Early signs of heel pain are usually due to plantar fasciitis (see pages 100–101). A heel spur develops when this pain is ignored and the chronic inflammation increases the stress on the fascia.

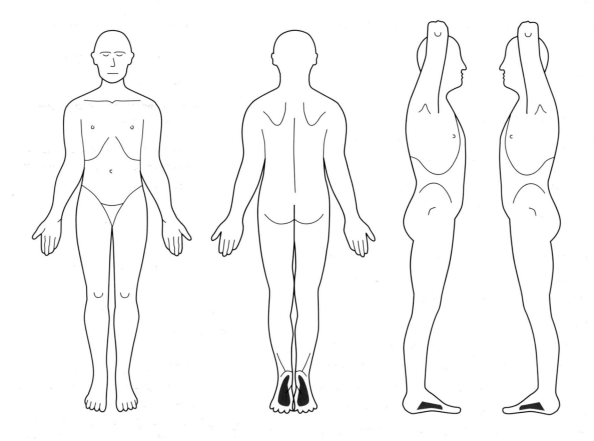

Aggravated by:	Eased by:
First steps in the morning	Activity/use
Beginning activity after a long rest	Ice
Start of a run/exercise	Massage

BLISTERS: TREATMENT AND PREVENTION

Causes
- Friction and irritation to the surface layer of the skin
- Moist, warm conditions of shoes and socks

Prevention
- Minimise friction
- Wear appropriate footwear
- Make sure your shoes are the right size and shape
- Wear socks made from synthetic blends
- Apply petroleum jelly or talcum power to your feet before running to reduce friction

Blister care
- Prevent the blister from growing and avoid infection.
- Small, unbroken blisters that are pain-free can be left alone to heal, as the best protection against infection is a blister's own skin.
- Large, painful blisters can be drained, but don't remove the top layer of skin. First, clean the blister with alcohol or soap and water. Then use a sterilised needle to puncture a small hole at the edge of the blister. Drain the fluid by applying gentle pressure. Put a bit of antibiotic ointment on the blister and cover with a plaster.
- If you are unsure, see a chiropodist/podiatrist to treat the blister for you.

TREATMENT TRAFFIC LIGHT

Self-treatment
- Recognise and treat plantar fasciitis early

Seek medical advice
- Tape the foot or use a heel cup
- Anti-inflammatory medication
- Specific exercises
- Physical therapy to try to reduce the inflammation
- A custom-made orthotic can control the abnormal stress and strain on the plantar fascia

Seek medical attention
- Cortisone injections
- If conservative therapy fails, surgery maybe indicated. Always consult a physiotherapist or physician for a thorough assessment and diagnosis.

ANKLE SPRAIN

Ankle sprains are the most common of all ankle injuries and occur when there is a stretching and tearing of the ligaments surrounding the ankle. You may also damage the other side of the ankle by bruising the bone. The most common cause of an ankle sprain is tripping when running on an uneven surface. The foot rolls in (inversion) or out (eversion) and the ligaments are stretched. Many of the problems resulting from sprains are due to blood and swelling in and around the ankle; therefore, it is important to minimise swelling as soon as possible.

SYMPTOMS

See below for areas of pain.

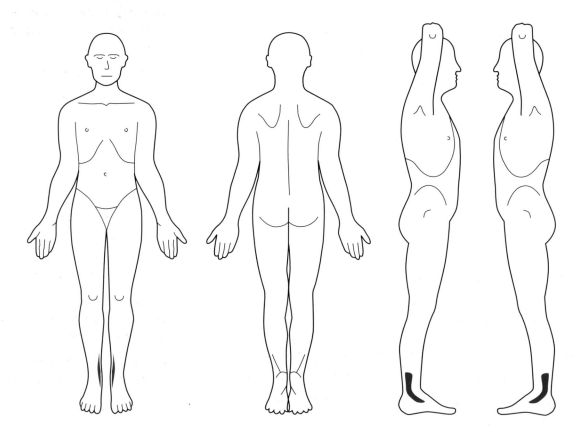

Aggravated by	Eased by
Weight-bearing	Rest
Moving the ankle	Ice
Touching the ankle	Compression
Walking	Elevation

Ankle sprains are classified by the degree of severity:

- Grade I: stretch and/or minor tear of the ligament without laxity
- Grade II: tear of ligament with some laxity
- Grade III: complete tear of the ligament.

Ankle sprains are often managed badly by runners as they are seen as a relatively minor injury. Even with a grade I sprain, it is important to ensure that you complete a full rehabilitation programme to reduce the risk of any further injury. With more severe sprains you will need to seek the advice of your physiotherapist and rule out the most serious injury, which is an avulsion, where the ligament has torn away from the bone.

PREDISPOSING FACTORS

- Previous ankle sprain
- Not completing rehab fully after a sprain
- Inappropriate footwear
- Running on uneven ground
- Muscle fatigue
- Poor balance and proprioception

ANKLE SPRAIN ACTION

Research has shown that the sooner you apply compression, ice and elevation, the sooner you will recover from your sprain. It is important to act quickly. Your main aim is to reduce as much swelling as possible.

TREATMENT TRAFFIC LIGHT

Self-treatment

- P.R.I.C.E.
- Range of motion exercises
- One simple exercise is to draw the letters of the alphabet with your toes
- Proprioception and balance exercises

Seek medical advice

- Gradually progress to full weight-bearing over several days as pain allows
- Tape the ankle to assist stability
- Mobilisation and stretches

Seek medical attention

- If you are unable to walk, see a physiotherapist to rule out serious injury; you may need crutches.
- Any ankle injury that does not respond to treatment in 1–2 weeks may be more serious.
- Always consult a physiotherapist for a thorough assessment and diagnosis.

ACHILLES TENDONITIS

The Achilles tendon is the largest and most vulnerable tendon in the body. It attaches the gastrocnemius and the soleus (calf) muscles of the lower leg to the heel. Tendons are strong but not very flexible so they can only stretch so far before they get inflamed, tear or, at worst, rupture. Achilles tendonitis is a chronic injury that occurs primarily from overuse. It tends to come on gradually until pain is constant and exercise is too painful to continue. The biggest cause of chronic Achilles tendonitis is ignoring early warning signs and pushing through pain.

SYMPTOMS

If the Achilles tendon is sore, or aches, you need to pay attention and rest it immediately. Other symptoms include crepitus, which is like a rubbing sensation and swelling. The tendon can also swell and become noticeably thicker than the tendon on the opposite leg. See below for areas of pain.

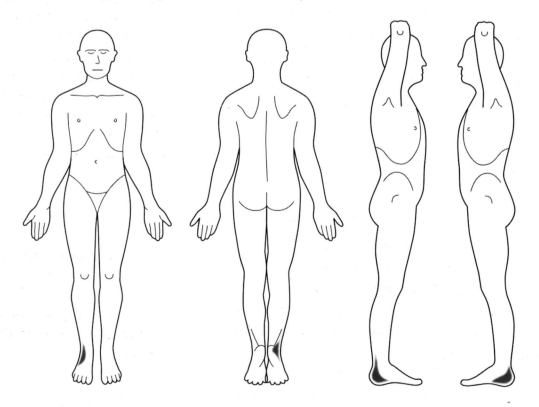

Aggravated by:	Eased by:
Walking	Rest
Weight-bearing	Ice
Touch	Anti-inflammatories

PREDISPOSING FACTORS

- Overuse
- Poor footwear
- Poor biomechanics
- Direct trauma
- Tight or weak calf muscles, which easily tighten and shorten when exercising, therefore increasing stress on the Achilles tendon
- Sudden increases in training, hill running or speed work

ACHILLES BURSITIS

You have more than 150 bursae throughout your body. These are little pouches of fluid that cushion movement and limit friction between bone and muscles or tendons. Bursitis is inflammation of a bursa. Inflammatory problems affecting your Achilles tendon, such as bursitis and tendonitis, often improve with home treatment and physiotherapy.

TENDON RUPTURE

At the time of tendon rupture you will hear a pop or snap, followed by an immediate sharp pain in your ankle and calf that makes it impossible to walk properly. It can feel like you have been kicked. Pain and swelling in your heel and an inability to bend your foot downward or walk normally signal that you may have ruptured your Achilles tendon. With a partial rupture, you may still be able to move your foot and you may experience only minor pain and swelling. An Achilles tendon rupture usually requires surgical repair.

TREATMENT TRAFFIC LIGHT

Self-treatment

- P.R.I.C.E.
- Reduce your training
- Stop speed training and hill running
- Gentle calf stretching; excessive stretching could aggravate the problem
- Post-exercise ice may also help

Seek medical advice

- Electrotherapy or acupuncture can be helpful for pain and swelling
- Strengthening the calf muscle can help reduce the stress on the Achilles tendon
- It is not necessary to stop activity completely (consider cross-training) as long as you pay attention to muscle soreness and reduce activity accordingly
- Heel raises or orthotics may be helpful

Seek medical attention

- If you are unable to walk, see a physiotherapist to rule out serious injury; you may need crutches.
- Always consult a physiotherapist for a thorough assessment and diagnosis.

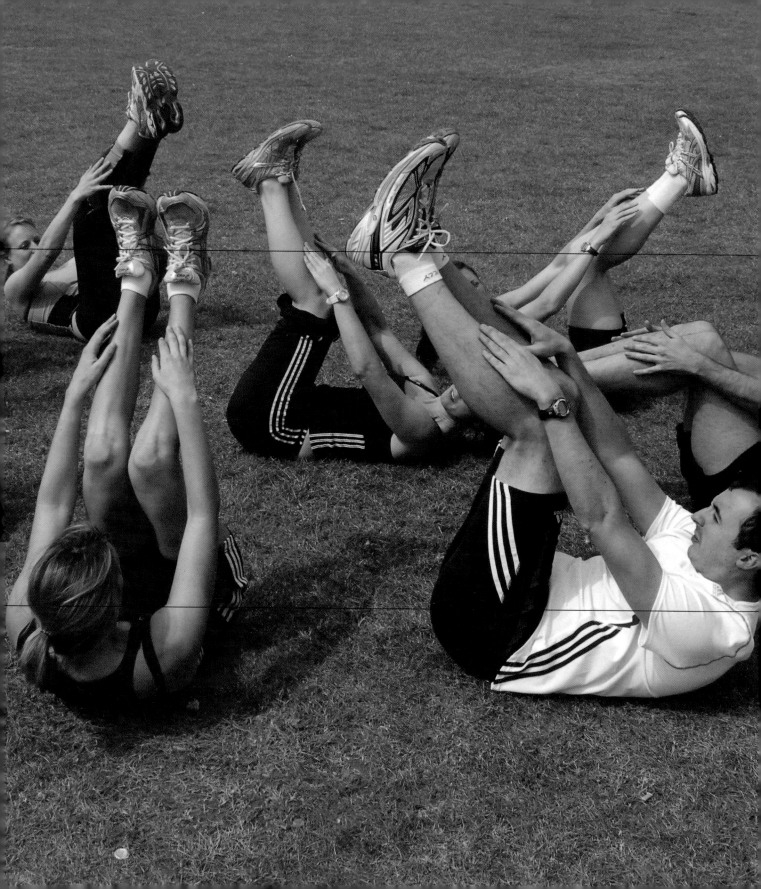

3

REPAIR AND PREVENTION

Now that you know what you've injured, or have identified areas for improvement in your MOT, the real work must begin.

You can't change the body type you were born with, but you can make the most of the body you have – keep it in good condition and you will be less likely to pick up an injury. I can't stop you tripping over any more than I can stop you crashing your car, but I don't need to be a mechanic to tell you that maintaining your car keeps it running.

In Part 3, you'll find stretches and strength-conditioning exercises which have worked for my running clients over the years.

CONTENTS

YOUR REPAIR AND PREVENTION PROGRAMME

The majority of runners who end up at the physiotherapy clinic have no idea how weak or tight some of their muscles are, but it is these weaknesses and imbalances that often lead to injury. The reason for this is that most runners spend all their training minutes and hours running, with little or no regard for stretching and strength conditioning. Most runners who do spend some precious minutes a week on strength and conditioning exercises have learned to do so the hard way – after being injured. Whether you are one of these people, or one of the smart ones who has decided to spend some quality time on prevention rather than cure, below you will find some stretches and exercises to get you into tip-top shape. After all, to keep the motoring analogy going, you have to service your car if you want it to work to its best ability.

Before you start using the exercises, there are a few things you need to know.

WHEN AND HOW OFTEN?

As mentioned earlier in the book, there are plenty of books and websites that tell you how to plan and schedule your running programme. However, it is worth mentioning a few things about when you should factor your stretching and strength-training sessions into your routine and how many exercises to incorporate.

There are many exercises to choose from in the following pages, but if you choose too many you will never get through them all. To help you choose which will be most specific to you, think back to the answers you gave in your service history and MOT questionnaires (see pages 23 and 26, respectively). Current and past injuries will reveal where you have tightness or muscle imbalances, and videoing yourself running will show up technique pointers to work on. As a guide, choose between two and four exercises per area depending on how many areas you need to work on. It may help to concentrate on different areas on different days, just as you do with your running sessions, so you can balance out the work on your body. This will also allow you to mix strength, conditioning and stretching with your running schedule. In addition, it is always wise to change your routine every four to six weeks by substituting one exercise for another; this allows you to concentrate on the same area, but challenges you and prevents you getting bored. One option is a rolling programme of exercises that are interchangeable over a few months. Remember, your stretching should remain a consistent part of your programme to allow you to maintain your new-found flexibility. This will of course vary depending on whether your routine was part of a recovery from injury programme, or a preventative-conditioning programme.

ACTIVE REST

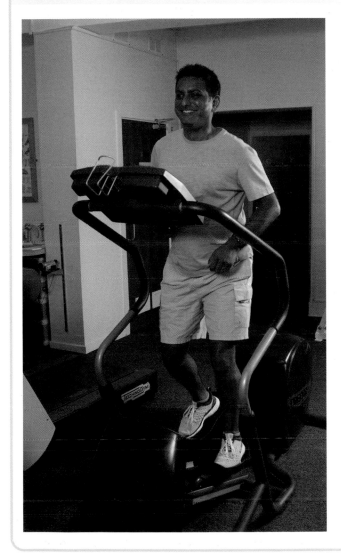

Active rest is a great way to maintain fitness when you are injured and can't run. It works by replacing a run with a session on the elliptical trainer, a swim or any low-impact activity. You can also think of your cool-down as a form of active rest that will hasten recovery after training. Just 10–15 minutes of light jogging and dynamic stretching can make all the difference and help to boost your recovery immediately. If you don't cool down, it can take up to four hours to completely clear the metabolic waste from your muscles. Stretching aids this process of removal, as well as helping to restore the muscles to their normal length.

Active rest can be used to describe your warm-up, injury training or short runs in between fast or long ones. Light activity will speed recovery faster than complete rest in most cases, the exception being when you have a serious injury that requires rest.

RUNNING SURFACES

Running on hard surfaces like roads is sometimes unavoidable, but you should make an effort to run on a variety of surfaces to reduce the mechanical shock to your joints and tendons. Soft surfaces such as grass or sand may tire your muscles more quickly and divots and pot-holes increase the risk of injury, but it is good for your body to feel variations and learn to adapt to different conditions. Sometimes the risk of injury has to come with the instruction to just be careful!

Treadmill running has a much lower impact than road running and is the perfect way to start running or get back to running after injury. It is also easier on your gluteal muscles (the muscles in the bottom that extend the hip) as the belt moves under your feet rather than you having to push yourself along outside. For even less impact the elliptical trainer is ideal, as you can mimic all the actions of running without any impact at all. Many of my injured marathon runners replace their long runs with sessions on the elliptical trainer so they maintain the endurance aspect while taking active rest from running.

WARMING UP

The benefit of a warm-up and a cool-down – whether for a run or a strength-training session – is a much debated issue, with many runners believing that they are unnecessary. In my experience, the lack of an effective warm-up, stretching and cool-down is a risk factor when considering running injuries. I really believe that these are more important than you might think.

Most athletes perform some type of regular warm-up and cool-down during training and racing, and we can learn much from this. A proper warm-up will increase the blood flow to the working muscles, which helps the muscles feel less stiff – this alone reduces the risk of injury and improves performance. Additional benefits are physiological and psychological preparation for what you are about to do. Bear in mind that the perfect warm-up is a very individual process that can only come with practice, experimentation and experience. Try warming up in various ways and at various intensities until you find what works best for you.

THE TEN PER CENT RULE: IMPROVE PERFORMANCE WITHOUT RISKING INJURY

It doesn't matter if you are new to running or training for your 10th marathon; it is essential to progress training at the right pace to meet your goals to avoid injuries. Increasing the intensity, time or pace during training is a common reason for injury. The ten per cent rule is an easy way to help both experienced runners and beginners avoid injury, yet still see continual improvement in performance.

- Once you know you are fit to start training safely, the main thing to remember is that you need to start and progress slowly.
- Following the ten per cent rule sets a limit on how much you can increase your training each week.
- Increase your running by **no more** than ten per cent each week. That includes distance, intensity, pace and time of exercise.
- If you haven't exercised for some time, a five per cent increase per week may be much more comfortable. If you are unsure of your ability, you can increase even slower.

To effectively improve your ability using the ten per cent rule, you must continue running from week to week. It can be a great motivator for new runners to get started, as well as for those who are preparing for a specific event.
For example:

WEEK 1	WEEK 2
2 miles	2.2 miles
5 miles	5.5 miles
10 miles	11 miles
20 miles	22 miles

All these distances can be used for running or a run-walk programme depending on your ability.

BENEFITS OF A PROPER WARM-UP

- Increased muscle temperature – a warm muscle will contract more forcefully and relax more quickly. The probability of overstretching a warm muscle and causing injury is far less than that of a cold muscle.
- Increased body temperature – this improves muscle flexibility and reduces the risk of strains.
- Efficient cooling – by activating the sweating mechanisms in the body, you can stay cool and help prevent overheating early in the training session or race.
- Improved range of movement – the range of motion in a joint is increased.
- Hormonal changes – your body increases its production of various hormones that regulate energy production. During a warm-up, the balance of these hormones makes more carbohydrates and fatty acids available for energy production.
- Mental preparation – the warm-up is also a good time to prepare mentally for a race, by clearing the mind and increasing focus. Positive imagery of you crossing the finish line will relax you and build concentration.

STRETCHING

Why should we stretch? The main reason for stretching is to ensure a full range of movement at the joints while maintaining extensibility and elasticity in the muscles. If a muscle becomes short or tight, the function and movement at a joint can be affected. By stretching, you will help to maintain the optimum and functional length in a muscle and in turn maintain or increase the amount of movement available in your joints. I can't promise that stretching will prevent injury outright, but it will prevent tightness and the muscle imbalances that are so commonly part of the presentation when someone is injured.

There are two ways to stretch – static and dynamic – and both ways are as helpful as they are different. The difference between the two is simple: dynamic stretching allows movement as part of the stretch, while in static stretching a position is maintained with the muscle in tension. I feel that you can get a better increase in range of motion with a dynamic stretch, but the choice depends on which part of the body you are trying to stretch and if you want to stretch during your training session or at the end. Each method has its benefits, so combining both into your routine will allow you to listen to your body and see which works best for you. On pages 116–159, you will see the stretches for each area of the body alongside the exercises for the area. This will help you to stay focused on the specific areas that you need to work on rather than adding lots of non-specific stretches into your routine.

How long you should hold a stretch is an area of debate and everyone will have a different time scale. Generally, people don't hold stretches for long enough, so doubling the time you hold your current stretches for will lead to a noticeable improvement in your flexibility; however, the rule of thumb from research is 30 seconds. You may need to stretch for longer and continue over a longer period of time before you see an improvement if you are recovering from an injury.

STRENGTH CONDITIONING

Strength conditioning is an important part of your training because it benefits your muscles directly and will help to prevent injury. The stronger you are, the better your ability to minimise the repetitive effects of running and maintain stable and aligned biomechanics.

Should I use weights?

You can use weights, but you don't have to; it depends on where and how you like to train. If you use a gym, working with weights will be easy; if you don't use a gym, it will be just as easy to train using your own body weight as resistance. Many people worry that using weights will build bulk, but this will only happen if you change your diet and train to a high-weight/low-reps regime. Working with weights will make you lean and strong so give it a try – you might like it. If you don't, that's fine too – this section of the book contains exercises that don't use weights but are just as effective.

What is meant by sets and reps?

Sets and reps are common terms used to explain how much training you have to do in a session. Sets are made up of reps (repetitions), which refers to the number of exercises you will be doing in one set. You can increase or decrease the number of reps to accommodate the session and what else you have done in the week.

HEAD AND TRUNK
THE ARMPIT SNIFF

TARGETS
Upper trapezius and scalene muscles in the neck.

SETS/REPS/TIME
1 set of 3 reps, little and often throughout the day.

HOW TO DO IT
This is a gentle stretch to muscles that can become tight when you are training or through poor posture.

1. Turn your head to the left.
2. Drop your chin down to look at your armpit.
3. Breathe in gently. As you breathe out, lower your nose closer towards your armpit. Hold for 10 seconds, relax the stretch for 2 seconds and repeat twice more. Stretch both the left and right sides.

TIP
To make this stretch more comfortable, take gentle steady breaths throughout.

VARIATION
Once you are familiar with this stretch it will become easier. To increase the stretch, gently over-press with your hand.

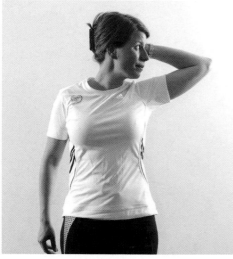

Fig. 3.1a Start position

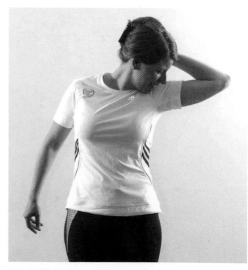

Fig. 3.1b End position

CHIN TUCKS

TARGETS

Mobilises the joints and loosens the muscles at the base of the neck and the upper thoracic spine.

SETS/REPS/TIME

1–2 sets of 10 reps, little and often.

HOW TO DO IT

This is a great exercise for stiff necks and poor postures, and you don't always have to be in the gym to benefit.

1. Sit up straight or lie on your back with your head supported.
2. Drop your chin slightly and keep your head in this position.
3. Gently push the tip of your tongue into the roof of your mouth.
4. If you are sitting down, move your head backwards; if you are lying down, push into the supporting surface, until you feel like you have a double chin.
5. Hold for 2–3 seconds, then relax your tongue and your double chin.

TIP

Never push into pain; keep it slow, gentle and controlled at all times.

VARIATIONS

- Lie on the floor with a firm pillow under your head and push your head into it, giving yourself a double chin. Slowly turn your head from side to side, maintaining the push backwards into the pillow. Your head should be in a comfortable position. Keep your knees bent for comfort. Repeat 3–5 times.
- Work against resistance and push your head into a gym ball.

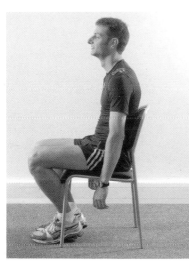

Fig. 3.2a Start position

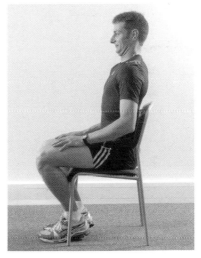

Fig. 3.2b End position

Case Study 1: Neck pain

Diagnosis:

Adaptive Postural Pain

Problem:

A 42-year-old man and novice runner presented with neck and shoulder pain. Onset was gradual, worsening over a 6-week period after starting running as a way to lose weight. His symptoms were intermittent but persistent, affecting his running, sleep and ability to read and work at a desk. He complained of muscle tightness around his neck and shoulders that affected his movement.

What makes it worse?	What makes it better?
Running	Painkillers
Reading	Massage
Computer work	Hot shower
Turning the head from side to side	

On assessment:

- Reduced range of movement in neck
- Poor posture and breathing pattern when running
- Tightness in the upper trapezius muscle
- No neurological signs or referred pain
- Overweight
- Poor general fitness, diet and fluid intake

Muscle strength:

Generally de-conditioned.

Acute care:

Recognise the need to investigate the cause of the pain.

Physiotherapy treatment and advice:

1. Acupuncture.
2. Manual therapy to improve neck movement.
3. Dynamic stretches to neck and shoulders.
4. Ergonomic assessment of workstation.
5. Cross-training for general cardiovascular fitness.

Self-management:

1. Develop structured run/walk programme.
2. Train to match current ability, gradually increasing as fitness improves.
3. Massage/self-massage and heat packs to reduce tension in tight muscles.
4. See dietician for healthy eating plan.
5. Have training plan that includes running, strength and conditioning.
6. Make lifestyle changes to improve health and posture awareness.
7. Core stability muscle activation and strength and conditioning training.

Lessons to learn:

1. Recognising the need to get fit can prompt major lifestyle changes.
2. New or returning runners will have to adapt to new mechanical stresses, which can cause problems if not taken slowly.
3. Desk-based jobs and a poor running posture may increase the risk of strain/injury.
4. Bad breathing patterns when running will overuse the muscle at the front of your neck, causing tension in other neck muscles.

Results:

This man attempted a running programme with the drive and training he was capable of at 20, not realising his true fitness level. The most important part of his treatment was to start a run/walk training programme that was equal to his ability (see pages 34-9. Treatment with acupuncture, manual therapy and heat packs helped to reduce the muscle spasm, allowed normal movement, and enabled the neck to relax at night so he could sleep. Changes were made to his general posture, particularly when sitting at his workstation (see page 119). Improvement was rapid; he was soon running with good posture and correct breathing. Running drills were specific to his running goal and assisted his strength and conditioning while avoiding injury.

He completed the London marathon in 2007 after losing 4 stone and improving his overall fitness.

GRANNY PRESS-UPS

TARGETS

Triceps and glutes.

SETS/REPS/TIME

Beginner: 3 sets of 10 reps; **intermediate**: 3 sets of 20 reps; **advanced**: continuous press-ups for 1 minute.

HOW TO DO IT

This is a great exercise for strengthening your arms and improving your arm swing. When your legs feel tired, pump those arms and you will keep on running!

1. Lie on your stomach with your arms in front of you and your fingertips touching.
2. Squeeze your buttocks (this will help to protect your back from an extension overstrain).
3. Slowly push up on your arms and then lower your chest back to the floor.

VARIATION

Try doing the same number of reps but much more slowly – this will really make your arms tired!

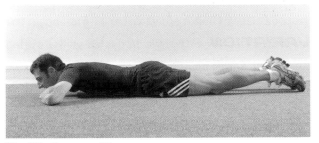

Fig. 3.3a Start position

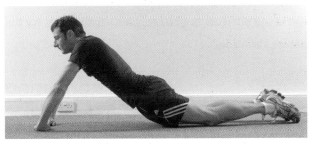

Fig. 3.3b End position

PROTECT YOUR POSTURE

Anyone who sits at a computer should know the benefits of having a good workstation setup. It never fails to surprise me how badly some people have to sit all day, every day. Compare your workstation with the one in Fig. 3.4 and make the changes needed to improve your desk. Avoiding postural aches and pains will help keep you in a state of 'permanent recovery' and will also help your running posture no end.

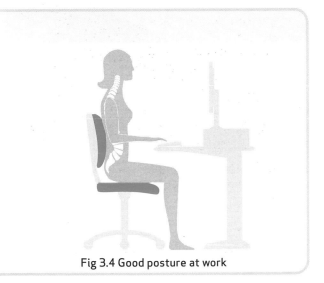

Fig 3.4 Good posture at work

Case Study 2: Low-back pain

Diagnosis:

Mechanical low-back pain

Problem:

A 35-year-old man who is an experienced runner presented with low-back pain. Onset was gradually worsening as he increased his running distance from 5km to 10km. Symptoms were intermittent and varied between an ache and a sharp pain when standing from a chair.

What makes it worse?	What makes it better?
Sitting to standing	Rest
Running	Changing posture
Putting socks on	Anti-inflammatories

On assessment:

- Reduced range of movement in the spine
- Tenderness in the lumbar spine on palpation
- Intermittent muscle spasm when moving
- No neurological signs or referred leg pain
- A neutral hip, knee and foot position
- History of previous episode of low-back pain

Muscle strength:

Weak, poor activation of core abdominal muscles, weak gluteals.

Acute care:

1. Stop running. Replace with cross-training on the elliptical trainer.
2. Use non-prescription painkillers and anti-inflammatories.
3. Reduce training to protect the injury.
4. Rest and ice to reduce muscle spasm.

Physiotherapy treatment and advice:

1. Acupuncture.
2. Exercises to strengthen the gluteals when standing.
3. Core stability training.
4. Balance work with a gym ball.
5. Manual therapy.
6. Dynamic stretches to the spine and hamstrings.
7. Running drills with core muscle activation.

Self-management:

1. Gradually increase training and running distance.
2. Have a training plan that includes running, strength and conditioning.
3. Core stability muscle activation, strength training and functional exercises.
4. Physiotherapy back classes or Pilates classes.

Lessons to learn:

1. In 95 per cent of cases, back pain is mechanical in nature and related to poor posture. How it is managed will dictate how well you recover and manage subsequent episodes.
2. It is crucially important to rehabilitate core muscles, making the exercises part of your strength and conditioning routine.
3. Do not take to your bed. Total rest may be necessary if the pain is severe, but active rest is more beneficial, having minimal impact on your fitness.

Results:

Acupuncture and painkillers helped to reduce the muscle spasm and allow normal movement, so that reduced impact exercise was possible. The most important part of rehabilitation was core stability training. He is running again after a long fight.

PIRIFORMIS STRETCH

TARGETS

The piriformis and glutes.

SETS/REPS

3 × 30-second holds.

HOW TO DO IT

1. Lie on your back and bring your right knee to your chest, then pull your right foot towards your left shoulder using your left hand.
2. Bring your left knee towards your chest, rest your right ankle on your left knee and hold the back of your left thigh with both hands.
3. Gently pull your left thigh towards you.

TIPS

After 30 seconds, relax the tension for 5 seconds before you repeat the stretch. This will help you to get a deeper stretch.

VARIATION

You can also perform this stretch while standing: place your outer calf and knee on a high stool and let your knee fall out to the side, opening your hip and groin. Bend the standing leg and lean forward to increase the stretch.

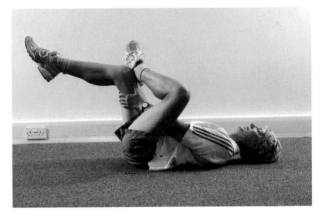

Fig. 3.11 Piriformis stretch

Case Study 3: Buttock pain (Piriformis syndrome)

Symptoms:

Pain, tightness, pulling, sciatica, pins and needles

Diagnosis:

Piriformis syndrome

Problem:

A 26-year-old woman presented complaining of buttock and leg pain. Onset of symptoms was gradual, but had become worse since training for a 10km race and increasing her speed-work. She has always suffered with tightness in her legs and admitted to not stretching enough. She cycles 5 miles a day, to and from work, and symptoms ease as she cycles, but tightness increases as the day goes on. She suffered from intermittent pins and needles in the leg when the pain was at its worst.

What makes it worse?	What makes it better?
Sitting/standing	Not running
Running	Changing position
Lying on the painful side in bed	Stretching

On assessment:

- Poor flexibility around the hip
- Poor balance on one leg
- Pain on palpation of the buttock
- Genu valgum (knock knees)
- Poor balance and proprioception
- Poor control of one-leg squat

Muscle strength:

Weak gluteals, poor core stability and poor general flexibility.

Acute care:

1. Need to investigate the cause of the pins and needles.

Physiotherapy treatment and advice:

1. Acupuncture.
2. Massage.
3. Proprioceptive and balance training.
4. Gait assessment and advice on the appropriate trainers.
5. Increase flexibility of the hip joints.
6. Running drills.

Self-management:

1. Dynamic stretch programme.
2. Need to change your training to address problems.
3. Improved strength and conditioning training - particularly in the gluteals.
4. Core stability training.

Lessons to learn:

1. Buttock and leg pain can be referred pain from the spine or the hip. A full assessment by a chartered physiotherapist is essential for correct diagnosis and subsequent management.
2. Overstretching when you have nerve pain from the spine can make things worse. You may need to work on other areas before you start to stretch.

Results:

It is crucially important to stretch: tight muscles can present as symptoms that mimic more serious conditions. Once reassured that nothing serious was wrong and treatment helped to ease the symptoms as stretching was added to her routine, progress was quick. An overhaul of her training programme and the addition of core stability and flexibility work improved her technique and abolished all symptoms.

BRIDGES

TARGETS

The glutes, adductors and core stability.

SETS/REPS

3 sets of 10 reps.

HOW TO DO IT

This exercise will strengthen your glutes and give you a butt to be proud of.

1. Lie on your back with your knees bent and your feet flat on the floor.
2. Place a cushion or medicine ball between your knees and hold it in place by squeezing your knees together.
3. Lift your pelvis off the floor and hold for 10 seconds, then release.

TIP

Squeeze a cushion between your knees until you can do it easily, then progress to a medicine ball.

VARIATION

Once you can do this easily, make it harder by following steps 1–3 but, once you have lifted your pelvis, extend one knee and then the other. Don't allow your pelvis to rock and keep the cushion or medicine ball in place.

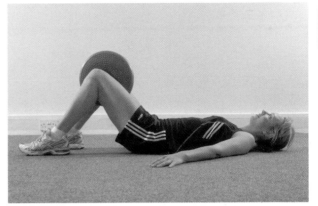
Fig. 3.12a Start position

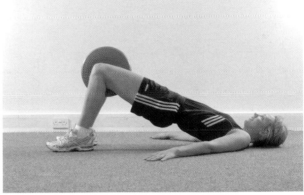
Fig. 3.12b End position

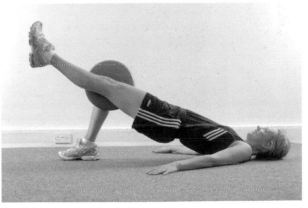
Fig. 3.12c Advanced position

ONE-LEGGED STEPPER

TARGETS

The glutes, quads and core stability.

SETS/REPS

2–5 minutes on each leg.

HOW TO DO IT

You will need a stepper to do this exercise, so it's definitely one for the gym.

1. Stand with one foot on the floor and the other on the stepper.

2. Making sure you maintain an excellent standing posture, slowly push the foot plate to the floor. As you push down, don't transfer your weight to push through the foot; keep your weight on the standing leg.

3. Raise your knee to the starting position and repeat.

VARIATION

This will be more difficult with increased resistance (the opposite to using a stepper with both feet) so to progress the exercise you will need to reverse the usual increased difficulty settings.

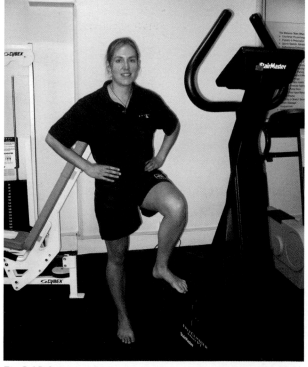

Fig 3.13 Start position

HIP DIPS

TARGETS
The core stabilisers, obliques and illiopsoas.

SETS/REPS
3 sets of 15 reps.

HOW TO DO IT
This will help to improve your core stability and single-leg balance, which are essential for running. The easiest variation is described, but you can follow the pictures for the alternative options.

1. Stand on one leg on the edge of a step with the other foot hovering above the floor.
2. With your hand on your hip, slowly reach the sole of your foot towards the floor.
3. The standing leg must stay straight as you lower the opposite leg and then bring it back to the starting position.

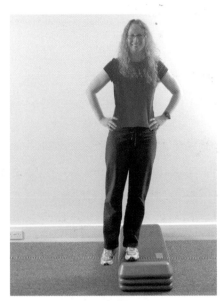

Fig. 3.14a Start position

TIPS
• Make sure you keep the standing knee straight; if you need help to balance hold on to a banister or wall.
• If you use a mirror, you will see the muscle on the side of your stomach lengthen if you are doing it correctly.

VARIATIONS
Use a gym ball under your knee or a piece of Theraband around your foot to add resistance.

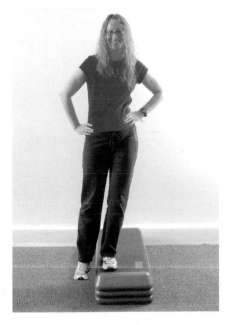

Fig. 3.14b End position

LEG CIRCLES

TARGETS

The glutes and your single-leg balance and stability.

SETS/REPS

6 sets of 10 reps.

HOW TO DO IT

This is a great exercise for your glutes and will help your alignment control in the leg.

1. Stand on one leg with the other leg lifted in front of you, 12 inches off the floor.

2. Circle your leg 10 times clockwise and then 10 times anti-clockwise. Don't put your foot to the floor.

3. Lift the same leg out to the side and again circle your leg 10 times clockwise and 10 times anti-clockwise. Don't put your foot to the floor.

4. Lift the same leg behind you and circle your leg 10 times clockwise and then 10 times anti-clockwise.

5. Repeat using the opposite leg.

TIP

Allow yourself to wobble; don't hold onto anything. If you feel you are about to lose your balance, circle your leg more slowly.

VARIATION

When you get very good at this, balance on a wobble cushion or a Bosue while performing the exercise.

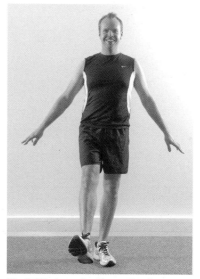

Fig 3.15a Leg circles to the front

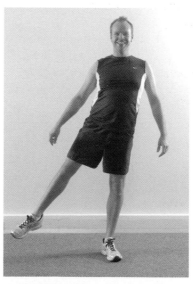

Fig 3.15b Leg circles to the side

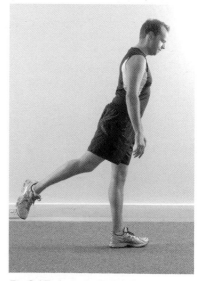

Fig 3.15c Leg circles to the back

COSSACK STRETCH

TARGETS

Hips, back, hamstrings, quads, adductors and glutes.

SETS/REPS

2 sets of 10 reps.

HOW TO DO IT

This is a real all-rounder and will save you time on stretching once you have mastered it as a drill. It's a great way to both loosen up before and cool down after a run.

1. Start with your legs wide apart and transfer your weight to one side into a lateral lunge position.

2. Balance your weight on the bent knee, keeping your heel to the floor and rolling the opposite hip outwards so that your toes face upwards and you feel the stretch in the back of the extended leg. Keep your groin at a 90-degree angle. Use your hands to keep you balanced.

3. Use your hands to help you turn your body into a deep lunge position so that you feel the stretch move from the hamstring to the front of the hip.

4. Turn the foot of the flexed leg outwards like Charlie Chaplin, then turn your body to follow the foot, keeping the other leg as straight as possible. You will feel the stretch move into your waist and upper hip on the straight leg and in your bottom on the side that is fully flexed.

TIP

Improve your flexibility with the dynamic hamstring and adductor stretches before you attempt this stretch, as it is an advanced drill.

VARIATION

You can vary this drill in so many ways to suit your current levels of fitness and flexibility. Break it up into individual stretches and master each in turn prior to using the drill as a sequence.

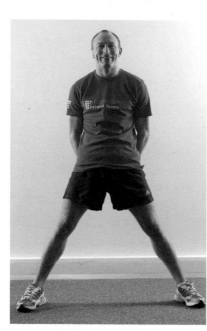

Fig. 3.16a Start position

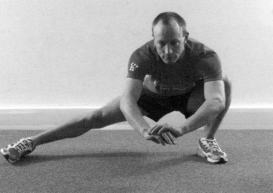

Fig. 3.16b Position two

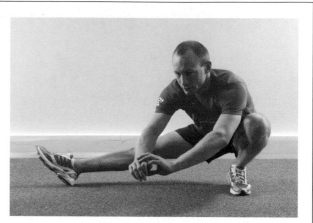

Fig. 3.16c Position three

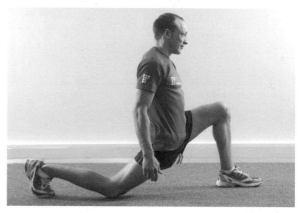

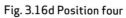

Fig. 3.16d Position four

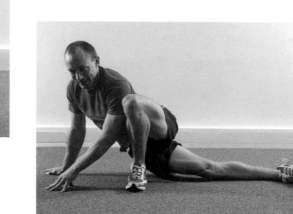

Fig. 3.16e End position

Case Study 4: Hip and thigh pain

Diagnosis:
Femoral stress fracture

Problem:
A 42-year-old woman who is an experienced runner presented with low-back pain and pain in the left groin, hip and thigh. At onset, pain was mainly in the hip and low back and no treatment really offered much relief. Pain was not severe enough to stop her running, but enough to seek assessment. She was increasing her training distances in preparation for the London marathon and was keen to continue. She was also running to help increase her bone density as a result of her osteoporosis.

What makes it worse?	What makes it better?
Walking	Rest
Moving the left hip	Painkillers
Sitting	
Bending forward	

On assessment:
- Previous foot fracture on the opposite leg.
- Low-back pain increasing with running greater distances.
- Stiffness in the lumbar spine and sacro-iliac joint.
- Poor flexibility in both hips.
- A neutral hip and knee position.
- Limping when walking.
- History of hypothyroidis and osteoporosis.

Muscle strength:
Weak gluteals, poor balance and poor single-leg control.

Acute care:
1. Referred to sport physician for X-ray and magnetic resonance imaging (MRI).
2. Review arranged with endocrinologist.
3. Need to rest and protect the injury.

Physiotherapy treatment and advice:
1. Acupuncture.
2. Gait analysis and re-education to gradually remove the need for crutches.
3. Rehabilitation to allow active rest and minimal-impact, pain-free exercise.
4. Progressive return to running on the elliptical trainer and treadmill.

Self-management:
1. Use non-prescription painkillers to reduce pain.
2. Proprioceptive exercises and running drills for the lower limb.
3. Positive mental attitude.
4. Resist the temptation to push too hard too soon.

Lessons to learn:
1. A serious injury like a femoral stress fracture can masquerade as a common sports injury.

Results:
Looking into the past medical history of this woman, there were three major clues suggesting that it was not a simple injury. A diagnosis of hypothyroidism and osteoporosis suggested issues with bone density, and previous fractures of the opposite foot may have led to an increased load on the injured side. The effect of muscular weakness in the glutes and poor control of single-leg squatting may have led to increased biomechanical stress and contributed to the stress fracture. A lack of flexibility in the hips and surrounding musculature was also a contributory factor. All of these are common in runners, but don't always result in a stress fracture.

She is now back to running outside. Minimal tightness around the hip is now the only symptom. It has taken 10 months to get to this stage of recovery, but she is progressing well.

DYNAMIC HAMSTRING STRETCH

TARGETS

Hamstrings, piriformis, tensa facilata and calf muscles.

SETS/REPS

10–20 reps in each position after every run.

HOW TO DO IT

This is one of the most effective ways to see a change in the flexibility of your hamstrings and your hips. It is a gentle way of stretching that is adjustable depending on how your legs are feeling.

1. Start by standing with your feet together, then take three small steps (heel to toe) so you stop with one foot in front of the other.
2. Lean forward and slide your hands down your leg to your ankle. The forward movement should come from your lower back and your hips.
3. Take three more small steps so your opposite foot is in front, and again reach your hands down to your ankle. Repeat 10–20 times.
4. The next stretch starts in the same way: take three small steps, but this time turn the toes of the front foot out, with the outer side of your heel level with the big toe of the back foot. Repeat 10–20 times.
5. The final stretch starts in the same way with three small steps. This time turn the front foot in, keeping the inside of your heel level with the big toe of the back foot.

TIP

Do not bounce or hold the stretch, just lean as far forward as you need to so you feel a stretch before returning to standing. It's the reparation of the movement that is important with this stretch, not how long you hold it.

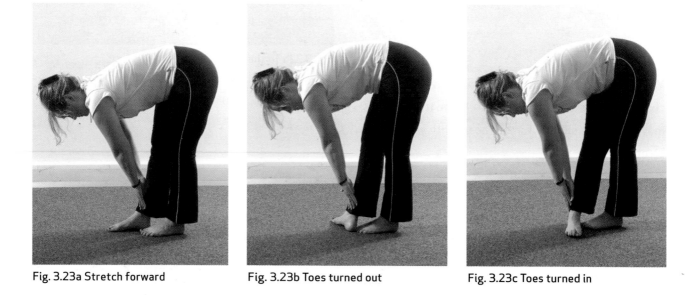

Fig. 3.23a Stretch forward   Fig. 3.23b Toes turned out   Fig. 3.23c Toes turned in

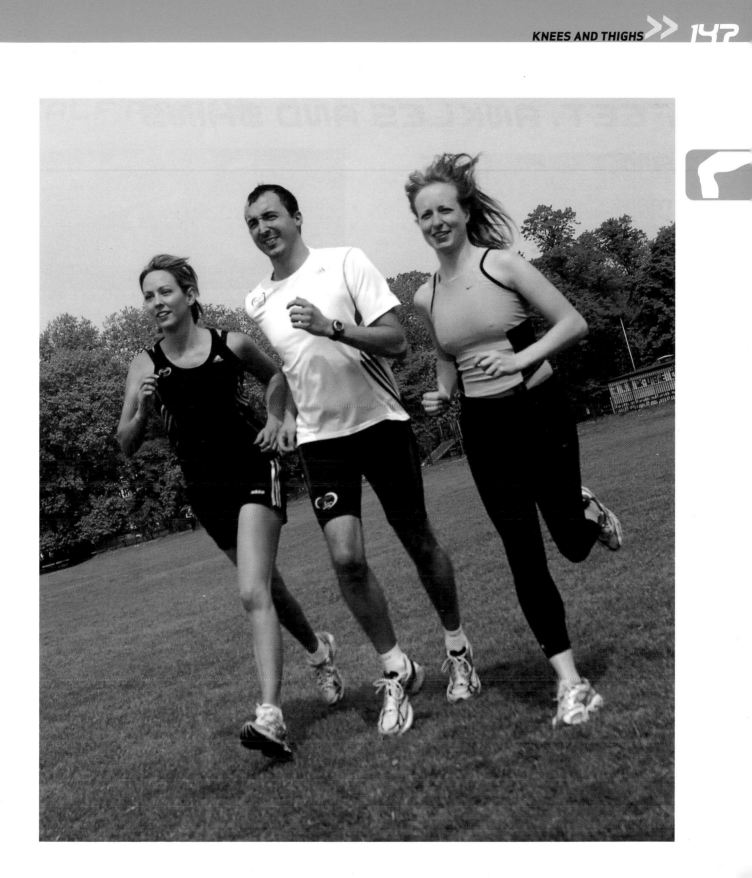

PRE-TIBIAL STRENGTHENING

TARGETS

The muscles of the shin.

SETS/REPS

2 sets of 15 reps.

HOW TO DO IT

This can look like you're falling over, but it will be worth it when you don't get shin splints!

1. Stand and balance with your weight on your heels.
2. Pull your toes up and towards your shins, then out to the side. Relax and repeat.

TIP

Having a wall behind you will help you to balance.

VARIATION

This exercise can also be performed sitting with a Theraband around your foot and fastened securely to a fixed point. Pull your toes up and towards you and then flick them out to the side.

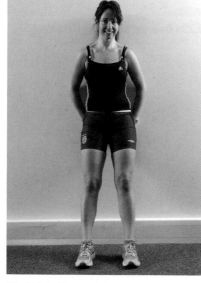
Fig. 3.30a Start position

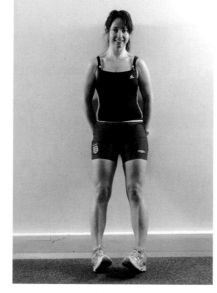
Fig. 3.30b Toes in

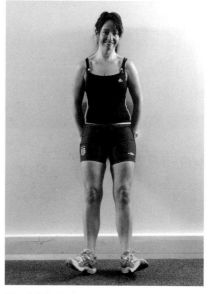
Fig. 3.30c Toes out

Case Study 10: Shin pain

Diagnosis:
Medial tibial stress syndrome (shin splints)

Problem:
A 34-year-old man presented complaining of shin pain. Initially, pain was severe when walking. He was unable to run, but was supposed to be in training for a marathon in 6 weeks' time. Pain started 2 weeks earlier and remained in spite of resting. He ran 18 miles even though a mild ache was present. He had no history of shin pain and was otherwise fit and well. He started training for the marathon after the death of his mother, raising money for the hospital where she died.

What makes it worse?	What makes it better?
Walking	Rest
Running	Ice
Pressure to the area	Painkillers

On assessment:
- A neutral hip and knee position
- Over-pronation of the forefoot
- Old trainers - a neutral shoe with minimal cushioning
- Tenderness on the shin bone when pressed
- Provocation on hopping

Muscle strength:
Normal

Acute care:
1. Need to rest and protect the injury.
2. P.R.I.C.E.

Physiotherapy treatment and advice:
1. Rule out stress fracture and compartment syndrome.
2. Taping to the shin to offload the area.
3. Orthopaedic walking book and crutches to reduce pressure and weight-bearing.
4. Gait analysis and advice on style of running shoe.
5. Ultrasound.
6. Acupuncture.
7. Massage.
8. Pre-tibial muscle strength training.

Self-management:
1. Gradually increase training distance.
2. Proprioceptive and balance training.
3. Training includes running, strength and conditioning.
4. Massage and stretches for muscle covering shin.

Lessons to learn:
1. Research the event and train properly for it. Management of your training programme is crucial.
2. If necessary, accept that you may have to undertake the marathon as a run/walk event to ensure reaching the finish line.

Results:
Pain was so severe on assessment that the priority was to rule out a stress fracture. Once ruled out, we had to resort to emergency measures. This is not what I advise for those wanting to run a marathon. In the 6 weeks prior to the race, he had to walk with crutches and he only ran twice on a treadmill - not an ideal training plan! This management was essential for a man who was determined to complete the distance in memory of his mum.

He completed the marathon without any serious injury, but prevention of injury and an appropriate training plan is a better way to achieve such an amazing goal.

SHIN STRETCH

TARGETS

The shin muscles and ankle dorsi-flexors.

SETS/REPS

3 sets of 30-second holds.

HOW TO DO IT

This is best performed on a soft surface such as a gym mat or even the bed.

1. Bend your legs underneath you. Sit on your heels. Lean back, placing your hands behind you.
2. You can point your toes behind you, towards each other or outwards to vary the stretch.
3. Put a towel under your feet to increase the stretch.

TIPS

If you have knee pain, this exercise is not one for you. See the variations below.

This is another good stretch to make part of your routine. You may be able to sit in this position as you dry your hair, eat your breakfast or do filing at work. Have a think about how you can fit it in to your routine without too much effort.

VARIATION

If you have trouble with your knees, try taking hold of your foot and resting your ankle on the opposite knee. Point your toes and hold your foot in this pointing position with your hands. Pull until you feel a stretch.

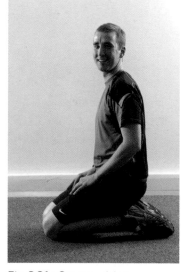

Fig. 3.31a Start position

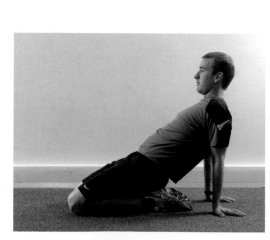

Fig. 3.31b End position

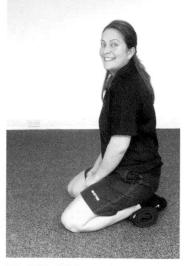

Fig. 3.31c With towel

THREE-WAY CALF STRETCH

TARGETS

The medial, lateral and central parts of the calf.

SETS/REPS

3 × 30 second hold in each position.

HOW TO DO IT

This is the classic calf stretch with a little more focus on each section of the calf muscle.

1. Stand facing a wall and place the ball of your foot against the wall, with your toes at 12 o'clock and your heel on the floor.

2. Lean into the wall to increase the stretch.

3. To stretch the lateral (outer) part of the calf, turn your toes to 10 o'clock and lean into the stretch.

4. To stretch the medial (inner) part of the calf, turn your toes to 2 o'clock and lean into the stretch.

TIP

As a rule of thumb, it is good to perform all three stretches, but if a specific part of your calf feels tight, focus on the stretch that targets that area.

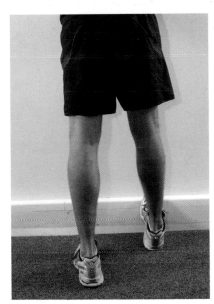

Fig. 3.32a Toes at 12 o'clock

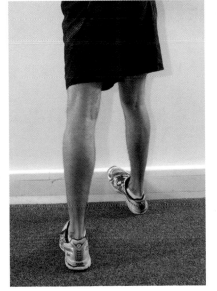

Fig. 3.32b Toes at 10 o'clock

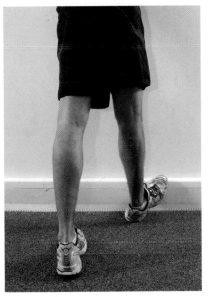

Fig. 3.32c Toes at 2 o'clock

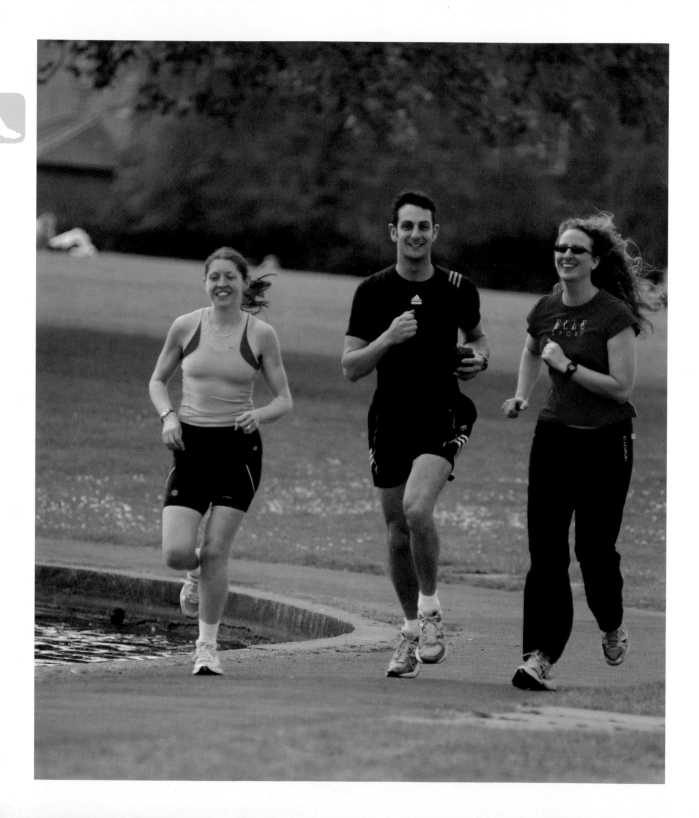

INDEX

ALSO AVAILABLE FROM A&C BLACK:

MARATHON: FROM START TO FINISH
SAM MURPHY (2004)
9780713668445   **£12.99**

You want to run a marathon, but you don't know where to start, how to train, what to eat and drink, how to dress, how to prepare for the race or, perhaps, even which race to do. *Marathon* guides you through the entire process: from your very first steps to beyond the finish line, ensuring that you not only complete your marathon but enjoy it, too!

MARATHON RUNNING (3rd edn)
RICHARD NERURKAR (publishing in 2008)
9780713688528   **£16.99**

Written by Britain's most successful marathon runner of the 1990s, this invaluable guide will help you get the most from your distance training. Covers everything you need to know, whether you're a complete beginner enchanted by the challenge of the London Marathon, or an experienced runner wishing to improve on racing strategy.

GET FIT: RUNNING
OWEN BARDER (2005)
9780713672046   **£9.99**

Get Fit: Running contains practical advice to help you buy the right gear, avoid injury, run safely, and improve fitness, with achievable training goals to keep you focused.

THE COMPLETE GUIDE TO STRETCHING (3rd edn)
CHRIS NORRIS (2007)
9780713683486   **£15.99**

The definitive practical guide for sports participants and recreational exercisers who are keen to achieve a level of flexibility to enhance their performance. Now in colour, fully updated and with brand new colour photographs, there are more than 70 exercises included to increase your range of motion right across the body.

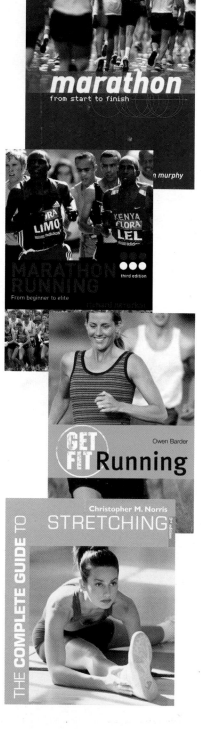